HAND PAIN
and Impairment

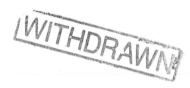

EDITION 3

HAND PAIN
and Impairment

RENE CAILLIET, M.D.

Professor and Chairman
Department of Rehabilitative Medicine
University of Southern California
School of Medicine
Los Angeles, California

 F. A. DAVIS COMPANY • Philadelphia

Also by Rene Cailliet:

LOW BACK PAIN SYNDROME
SHOULDER PAIN
NECK AND ARM PAIN
FOOT AND ANKLE PAIN
KNEE PAIN AND DISABILITY
SOFT TISSUE PAIN DISABILITY

Library of Congress Cataloging in Publication Data

Cailliet, René.
 Hand pain and impairment.

 Rev. ed. of: Hand pain and impairment. 2nd ed. 1975.
 Includes bibliographies and index.
 1. Hand—Diseases. 2. Pain. I. Title. [DNLM: 1. Hand.
2. Pain—Therapy. WE 830 C134h]
RC951.C24   1982   617'.575   82-2535
 ISBN 0-8036-1618-X   AACR2

PREFACE

Early evaluation and adequate treatment are necessary to the future normal functioning of the impaired hand. Too often, however, early evaluation and treatment are mismanaged because of the anatomic intricacy involved. Adequately informed, the primary physician—who may be a family physician, physiatrist, or internist—can reduce or avoid the need for reconstructive surgery, or at least allow the patient to face surgery with a salvageable hand.

This book provides the nonspecialist with information to better evaluate the impaired hand and initiate proper treatment. Therefore, the text is not exhaustive, and the presentation of the functional anatomy of the hand remains simplified. Although a simple explanation of a complex subject is possible, an easy understanding is not; it is hoped that this book will facilitate that understanding.

RENE CAILLIET, M.D.

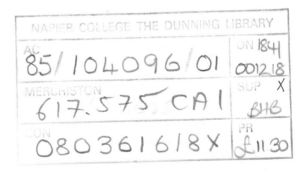
v

CONTENTS

ILLUSTRATIONS

xi

xiii

CHAPTER 1

Functional Anatomy

The hand is a complex machine, so intricate in its construction and function that great detail must be given to the discussion of its functional anatomy. The hand is an organ of grasp as well as of fine movements. It is an organ of sensation, fine discrimination, and exquisite dexterity. The large portion of the brain that controls the hand is evidence of the intricacies of this organ.

To understand disease and damage of the hand and its treatment, a basic knowledge of the normal hand is necessary. The primary role of the entire upper limb—shoulder, arm, elbow, forearm—is to place the hand in its proper position of function.

Restoration of function is the objective of treatment. Appearance, though important, is secondary. Early care is paramount, because ultimate reconstructive treatment too often leaves much to be desired. Because the hand tolerates immobilization poorly, the balance between immobilization and movement is a fine line requiring good clinical judgment. Whereas the wrist can be fully immobilized for many weeks and recover complete mobility, the hand and fingers cannot survive even brief immobilization.

ANATOMY

Wrist

The wrist joint is the articulation between the forearm and the carpal bones and is known as the carpus. The radiocarpal and radioulnar joints have mobility in many planes resembling a universal joint in man-made machines. The bones forming the carpal rows and their relationship to the radius and ulna are shown in Figure 1.

The distal end of the radius is concave. It usually reaches further distally on its radial than on its ulnar side, although in 60 percent of cases

1

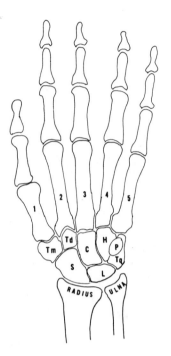

FIGURE 1. Bones of the hand. The composite of the bones of the *left* hand viewed from the palmar surface. The proximal row contains the (navicular) scaphoid (S), lunate (L), and triquetrum (Tq). The distal row contains the trapezium (greater multangular) (Tm), trapezoid (lesser multangular) (Td), capitate, and hamate. The pisiform (P) is considered to be in the proximal row.

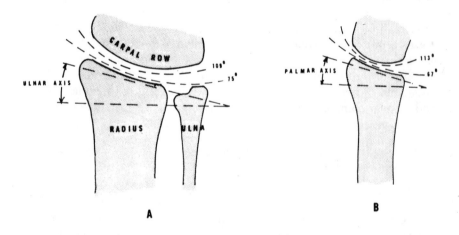

FIGURE 2. Relationship of the carpal row to the radioulnar surface. (A) The radial margin of the radius protrudes further than does the ulnar side. The articular surface is thus on an oblique plane. (B) The dorsal edge protrudes further than the palmar (volar) margin. The joint surfaces are incongruous; the carpal row is more convex than the opposing surface of the radius.

2

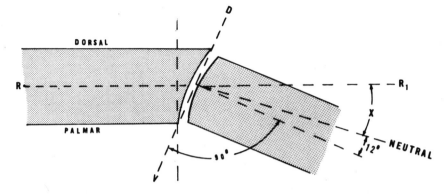

FIGURE 3. Wrist in neutral position. The *neutral* (resting) position of the wrist is slightly palmar and ulnar. Neutral is calculated as 12° of extension from plane perpendicular to the end of the radius DV and thus palmar to the axis of the radius RR_1. X is the degree of palmar flexion from the axis of the radius RR_1.

lengths are equal. The dorsal surface is longer than the palmar (Fig. 2B). This structural configuration causes the hand to rest in a slight ulnar and palmar posture (Fig. 3). The distal end of the ulna does not articulate with any carpal bones and can be surgically removed without impairing wrist motion.

The radioulnar surface is less concave transversely than anteroposteriorly. The curvature of the proximal carpal row is greater than the opposing curve of the radioulnar surface, viewed both dorsally and laterally (Fig. 2). The discrepancy of these two curves permits greater excursion of flexion-extension than radioulnar motion. The movements of the wrist are pictured in Figure 4: 80° flexion, 70° extension, 30° ulnar abduction, and 20° radial abduction. The greater degree of flexion (compared with extension) and of ulnar abduction (compared with radial abduction) is due to the angulation of the distal articular surface of the radius (see Fig. 2) and to the fact that the dorsal wrist ligaments are more slack than the palmar ligaments.

Motion of the radiocarpal joint essentially consists of flexion-extension and transverse (radioulnar) movements (see Fig. 4.) There is *no* rotation about the longitudinal axis. Pronation and supination of the hand thus occur exclusively at the proximal radioulnar articulation in the forearm. Normal range of pronation and supination as measured with the elbow flexed is 90° in either direction.

The wrist does not move in a direct plane (Fig. 5). Movement occurs along a plane between radial extension and ulnar flexion and an opposite plane of ulnar extension and radial flexion. These combined movements are related to the direction of the muscles and their tendons acting across the wrist.

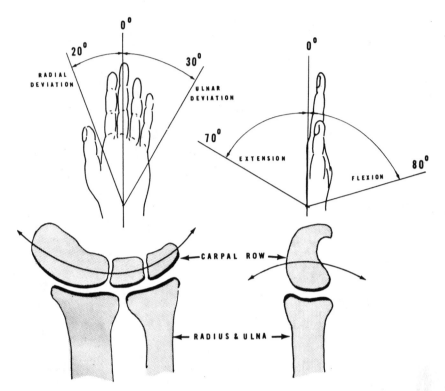

FIGURE 4. Range of wrist movement. Flexion-extension (dorsal-palmar) and lateral (radial-ulnar) are shown as an average. Neutral, as discussed in Figure 3, is not a true zero degree. No rotation occurs about the longitudinal axis.

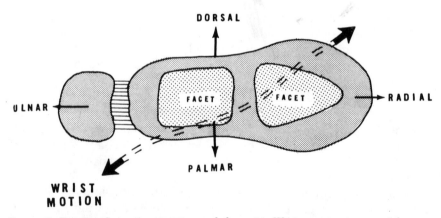

FIGURE 5. Functional movement patterns of the wrist. Wrist movements are not in one plane. All the muscles across the wrist act *obliquely*. Therefore, wrist movement is radiodorsal to ulnar-palmar. This plane of wrist movement is due to antagonistic muscle group pairing—extensor carpi radialis versus flexor carpi ulnaris and the long flexors of the fingers.

All the muscles of the hand originate primarily in the forearm and pass over the wrist and carpal bones to insert into the digits. No muscle inserts into any carpal bone other than the flexor carpi ulnaris to the pisiform. The muscles cross the radiocarpal, midcarpal, and carpometacarpal joints to attach upon the metacarpal and phalangeal bones. These tendons control the joints they traverse.

As noted in Figure 5, there are two facets on the radius. The lateral facet is triangular and articulates with the scaphoid bone and the medial is cuboid and articulates with the lunate bone. A cartilage joins the distal end of the radius to the styloid of the ulna (Figs. 5 and 6). The movement of the carpal row upon the radius and the triangular ligament is that of *gliding* (see Fig. 6). As the hand flexes in a palmar direction, the carpal row glides dorsally. In radial abduction of the hand, the proximal carpal row glides in an ulnar direction. To permit this gliding motion the capsule must be elastic and the ligaments sufficiently lax.

The major functional ligaments of the wrist (Fig. 7) are essentially the longitudinal, radial, and ulnar ligaments, as well as the transverse and oblique ligaments located on the dorsal and palmar surfaces.

The ulnar collateral ligament arises from the styloid process of the ulna and the triangular cartilage and attaches to the pisiform. It becomes taut on radial abduction of the hand. The radial collateral ligament arises from the radial styloid process, attaches to the scaphoid, and passes on to the trapezium and the first metacarpal. It becomes taut with ulnar deviation of the hand.

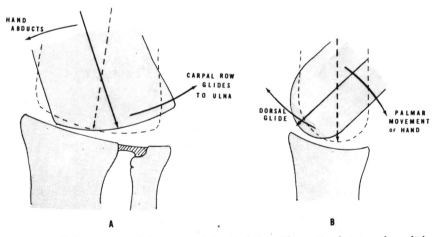

FIGURE 6. Gliding motion of the carporadial articulation. The motion between the radial surface and the proximal carpal row is that of gliding. The carpal bones glide in the direction opposite from the hand's movements. This gliding movement is permitted by capsular and ligamentous laxity.

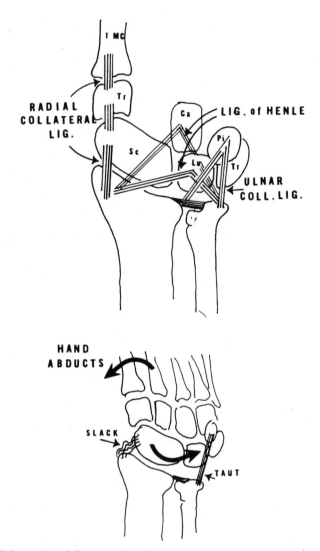

FIGURE 7. Ligaments of the wrist. The ulnar and radial collateral and the dorsal and palmar oblique ligaments support the wrist. Radial deviation of the hand tightens the ulnar collateral ligaments; ulnar deviation tightens the radial ligaments.

The transverse-oblique ligaments of the wrist on the palmar surface maintain the carpal arch. The palmar ulnar and palmar radiocarpal ligaments converge at the midline to attach to the lunate and capitate bones. This arcuate ligament is known as the ligament of Henle. The dorsal ligaments of the wrist are less symmetrical and more lax. Supination of the hand tightens the palmar ligaments, and pronation tightens the dorsal ligaments.

6

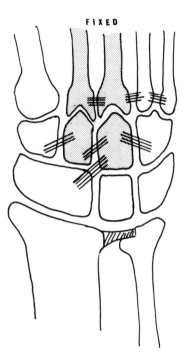

FIGURE 8. Intercarpal ligaments. The dorsal ligaments are related. The palmar ligaments shown here are transverse in their direction radiating principally from the capitate. There are few ligaments between the proximal and distal carpal rows.

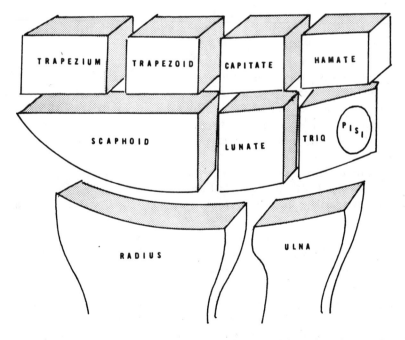

FIGURE 9. Carpal bones (schematic). The left hand is viewed from the palmar surface.

7

The intercarpal ligaments (Fig. 8) are placed to fortify the hand for any impact imposed upon the knuckles such as striking with a closed fist. The second and third metacarpals are fixed at their base and are immobile (see metacarpal section, this chapter). The strong intercarpal ligaments strengthen the fourth and first metacarpals by their attachment to this fixed central pillar. The obliquity of these intercarpal ligaments also permits movement of the carpal bones.

Carpal Bones

The eight carpal bones are arranged in two rows. Each is cuboid with six surfaces—four surfaces covered with cartilage to articulate with the adjacent bones and two surfaces (dorsal and palmar) roughened for ligamentous attachments.

The proximal carpal row (Fig. 9) contains the scaphoid, lunate, and triquetrum. The pisiform is the fourth carpal bone in the proximal row but it is placed on the palmar surface of the triquetrum and is considered a *sesamoid* bone. The proximal carpal row articulates with the radius and the triangular cartilage to form the wrist joint.

The distal carpal row contains the os trapezium ([NA] greater multangular bone), os trapezoideum ([NA] lesser multangular bone), capitate, and the hamate. The distal border of the proximal carpal row is concave and the proximal border is convex. The trapezium and trapezoid articulate with the scaphoid, the capitate with the lunate, and the hamate with the triquetrum (see Fig. 9).

In radial abduction of the hand, the proximal row moves in an ulnar direction as does the distal row upon the proximal row (Fig. 10). The capitate glides ulnarly and approximates towards the proximal row causing a "close-packed" congruity. In ulnar deviation of the hand, the capitate moves towards the radial side and disengages from the proximal row. Of the carpal bones, the scaphoid moves the most—as much as one centimeter.

In palmar flexion and dorsal extension, the distal carpi glide upon the proximal carpal row. The greatest degree of wrist-palmar flexion occurs at the radiocarpal joint, but a significant degree occurs at the intercarpal joints. In summary:

1. Palmar flexion of the wrist occurs mainly in the radiocarpal joint and secondarily in the midcarpal joints.
2. Dorsiflexion (extension) occurs mostly in the midcarpal joints and secondarily in the radiocarpal joint.
3. Radial deviation occurs mostly in the midcarpal joints and ulnar deviation mostly in the radiocarpal joint.

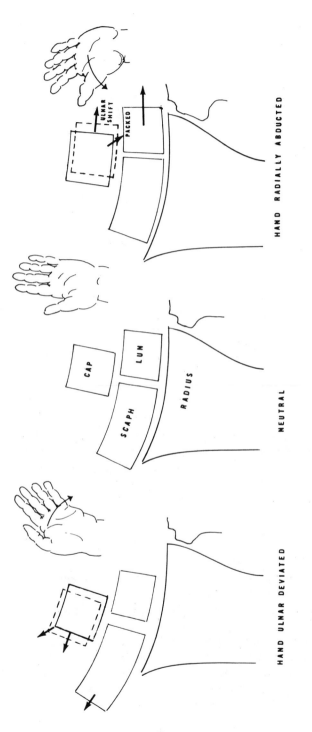

FIGURE 10. Carpal movement. When the hand moves radially, the carpal rows move in the opposite (ulnar) direction. The capitate glides ulnarly and *toward* the proximal row to pack tight. In ulnar movement of the hand, the opposite occurs.

9

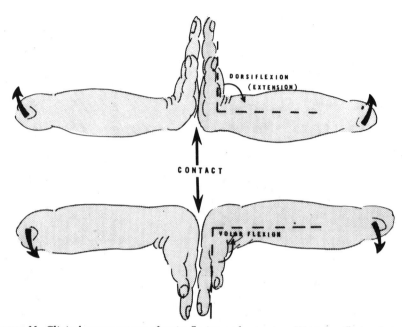

FIGURE 11. Clinical measurement of wrist flexion and extension. Wrist dorsiflexion (extension) can be estimated by placing the palms together and raising the elbows without allowing the palms to lose contact. Wrist palmar flexion can be determined by placing the backs of the hands together, fingers facing down, and then lowering the elbows until the hands begin to separate.

Clinically the degree of flexion-extension of the wrist can be accurately determined by placing the two hands together, palms and fingers touching, and raising the elbows (Fig. 11). Flexion range can be determined by placing the hands together, dorsal surface to dorsal surface, and lowering the elbows. Measurable limitation for recording requires measurement with a protractor.

Carpal Arch

The carpal bones form an arch that is concave on its palmar surface. The superficial ligament that spans this arch and maintains it, acting as a tie beam, is called the flexor retinaculum or the transverse carpal ligament (Fig. 12). This ligament is comprised of a proximal and a distal band.

The proximal band attaches from the tubercle of the navicular to the pisiform. Because the pisiform is movable, this band may be relaxed. The pisiform is essentially a sesamoid bone within the tendon of the flexor carpi ulnaris. The pisiform becomes "fixed" when this tendon is taut. The proximal band of the transverse carpal ligament becomes taut when the

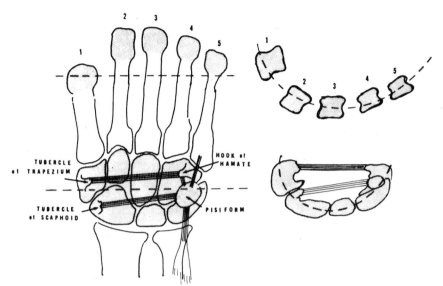

FIGURE 12. Transverse carpal ligament. Also termed the *flexor retinaculum*, this ligament bridges the arch of the carpal rows. It is formed by two bands—the proximal extending from the tubercle of scaphoid to the pisiform, and the distal band from the tubercle of the trapezium to the hook of the hamate.

flexor carpi ulnaris is contracted (Fig. 13), that is, when the hand is firmly held in an ulnar flexed position. The distal band of the transverse carpal ligament connects the tubercle of the trapezium to the hook of the hamate. Because these are fixed points, this band is always taut.

The concavity formed by the arched carpal bones spanned by the transverse carpal ligament is termed the *carpal tunnel* (Fig. 14). This tunnel would be deep enough to permit the entrance of a finger if all its contents were removed. The tunnel contains the tendons of the flexor digitorum profundus, which lie upon the carpal bones, and their connecting ligaments. Nearer to the surface is the layer of flexor digitorum superficialis tendons. Within the canal are also found the flexor carpi radialis tendon, flexor pollicis longus tendon, and the median nerve. The transverse carpal ligament restricts the "bowing" of the long flexor tendons of the fingers when the wrist is flexed and protects the median nerve from external pressure; it is also the site of origin of the thenar and hypothenar muscles.

The superficial landmarks of the structures on the palmar aspect of the wrist are shown in Figure 15. The distal skin crease of the wrist corresponds to the proximal border of the transverse carpal ligament. The flexor carpi radialis leads to the tubercle of the scaphoid and can be palpated when the clenched fist is flexed and radially abducted against resistance. The flexor carpi ulnaris leads to the pisiform and can be palpated when the clenched fist is flexed in an ulnar-deviated direction.

11

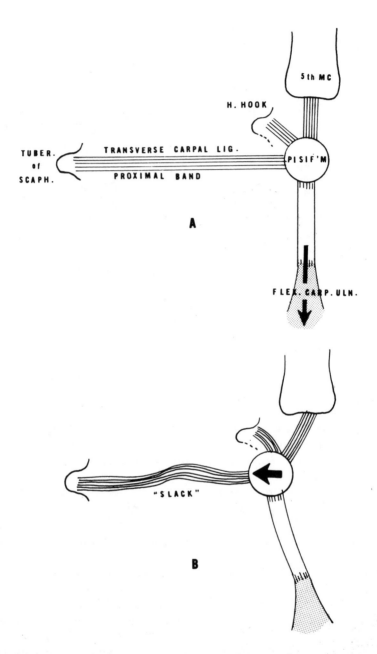

FIGURE 13. Proximal band of transverse carpal ligament. This structure is taut or slack depending upon the tension on the pisiform by the flexor carpi ulnaris. The pisiform is a sesamoid bone within the tendon of the flexor carpi ulnaris which attaches to the base of the fifth metacarpal and the hook of the hamate. (A) The contracted muscle tenses the transverse ligament. (B) Both are slack.

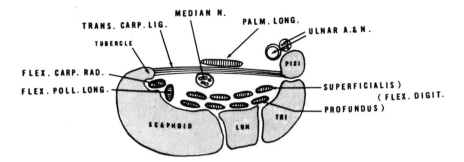

FIGURE 14. Carpal tunnel contents. The tunnel formed by the carpal bones and the spanning transverse carpal ligament contains the tendons of the long finger flexors (deep and superficial), tendons of the flexor pollicis longus and flexor carpi radialis, and the median nerve.

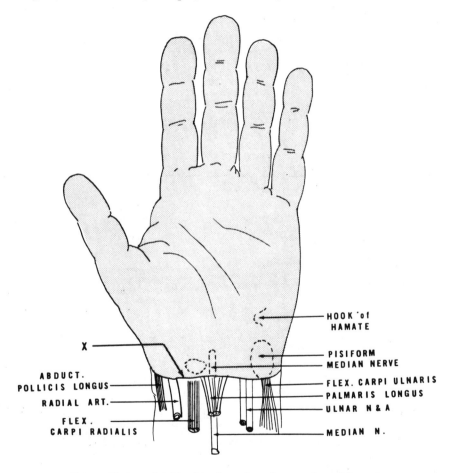

FIGURE 15. Superficial landmarks at the palmar surface of the wrist.

13

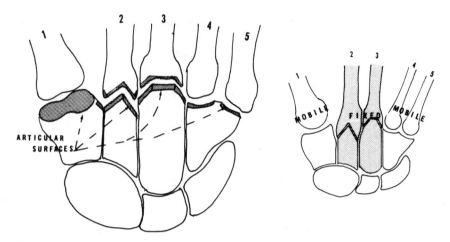

FIGURE 16. Carpometacarpal articulations. Five metacarpal bones articulate with four carpal bones. The second and the third metacarpal immobilize this segment by their numerous facets, close apposition of the planes of these facets, and the deep inset of the second metacarpal against the trapezoid and between the trapezium and the capitate. The first, fourth, and fifth metacarpals are mobile about this central fixed segment.

The median nerve cannot be palpated at the wrist. It lies under the palmaris longus tendon, which can be palpated and is seen in the midregion of the wrist when the clenched first is flexed in a midline position and against resistance.

The radial artery is palpable on the radial side between the tendon of the flexor carpi radialis and the abductor pollicis longus. The ulnar artery is palpable just to the radial side of the flexor carpi ulnaris tendon. The radial artery is readily palpable, but the ulnar artery is too deep under a thick fascia to be readily palpated.

Carpometacarpal Articulations

The distal border of the carpal bones is irregular. Four carpal bones articulate with five metacarpal bones. The fourth and fifth metacarpals articulate with two concave facets of the hamate (Fig. 16). The first (thumb) articulates with the saddle-shaped trapezium. The first, fourth, and fifth metacarpals have mobile joints. The second and third metacarpals form the immobile joints (Fig. 17). The second metacarpal has a gutter-shaped surface that fits over the central ridge of the trapezoid. The three protruding facets of the capitate are in direct contact with the three opposing facets of the third metacarpal. There is also a small facet of the third metacarpal in contact with the base of the second metacarpal. Being so wedged both the second and third metacarpals are immobile. In the *cupping* motion of the hand, the carpometacarpal joints move about this

14

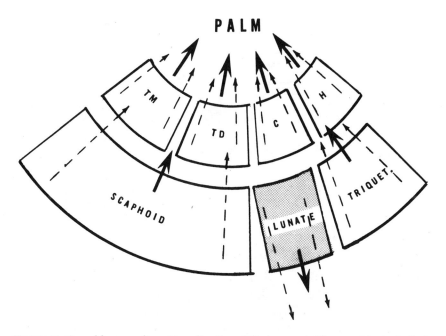

FIGURE 17. Carpal bone configuration, direction of displacement. The carpal bones by their shape form the palmar concavity and the dorsal convexity of the hand. The bones are broader on their dorsal surfaces and narrow on their palmar surface. This shape causes them to dislocate dorsally (with the exception of the lunate bone).

central immobile segment. The first metacarpal articulates on the radial side and the fourth and fifth (ring and little fingers) on the ulnar side of the "fixed" segment.

Metacarpophalangeal Articulations

The distal portion of the metacarpal is covered by hyaline cartilage that extends slightly over the dorsum and around the palmar surface on a rounded surface (Fig. 18). The ends are slightly flattened. Flexion-extension (dorsal-palmar), abduction-adduction, and some rotation (pronation-supination) are possible at this joint. Flexion-extension and abduction-adduction are voluntary motions but rotation is possible only as a passive motion.

The capsule of these joints is redundant to permit motion in which the concave surface of the phalanx *glides* along the convex surface of the metacarpal. The proximal surface of the phalanx has an arc of 20° whereas the metacarpal head has a surface arc of 180°. Motion of the metacarpophalangeal joint is 90° of palmar flexion and usually 20° of hyperextension (see Fig. 18).

15

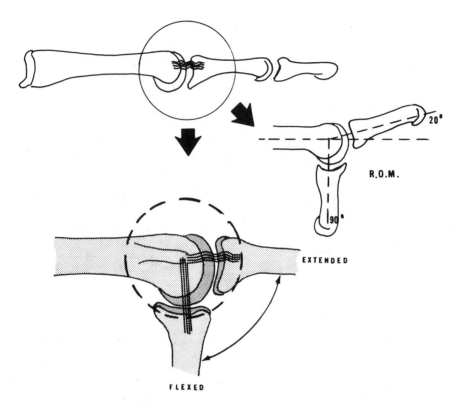

FIGURE 18. Metacarpophalangeal joints. As a result of the eccentric radius of rotation about the axis of the head of the metacarpal (dotted circle), flexion of the phalanx causes the collateral ligaments to become taut. The laxity of the ligaments in extension permits some lateral motion. Range of motion (ROM) is 90° flexion and 20° hyperextension.

Abduction and adduction of the metacarpophalangeal joint is limited when the finger is flexed because the head is flattened at its distal margin and the collateral ligaments are made taut in flexion. The collateral ligaments originate from a small tubercle eccentrically located on the lateral surfaces of the head. With the finger extended, the collateral ligaments are slack and permit lateral motion. In the flexed position, the base of the phalanx seats firmly against the surface of the metacarpal surface which now is further away from the axis of rotation. The ligaments thus become taut. On the palmar aspect of the joint the condyles are also broader than at the dorsal aspect which further tightens the ligaments.

There are no ligaments on the dorsal surface of the metacarpophalangeal joints. Here the limiting tissues are the extensor tendons of the fingers. The palmar aspect of these joints is reinforced by the *palmar plates* (Fig. 19). These are fibrocartilaginous plates in which the distal portion is cartilaginous and is firmly attached to the proximal portion of the pha-

16

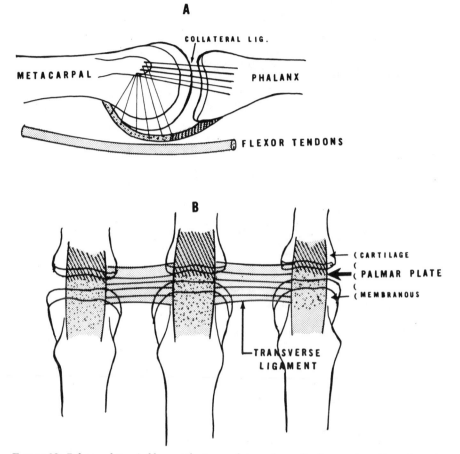

A

COLLATERAL LIG.

METACARPAL

PHALANX

FLEXOR TENDONS

B

(CARTILAGE

(PALMAR PLATE

(MEMBRANOUS

TRANSVERSE LIGAMENT

FIGURE 19. Palmar plate. A fibrocartilaginous plate replaces the ligament on the palmar surface of the joint. The plate is firmly held to the metacarpal by fibers of the collateral ligament. (A) The cartilaginous portion is firmly attached to the phalanx. (B) Palmar view shows the deep transverse ligament that connects the plates and prevents lateral motion of all the metacarpals except the thumb. The proximal membranous portion is loosely attached to the metacarpal.

lanx. The proximal portion of the plate is membranous and is loosely attached to the metacarpal.

The plates are held firmly against the joints by fibers of the collateral ligaments and are connected to each other by the deep transverse ligaments (Figs. 19 and 20). These plates reinforce the joint capsule and interpose between the joint surfaces and the flexor tendons that traverse the joint.

Subluxation of the metacarpophalangeal joint will often tear the plate from its metacarpal attachment. Because of the membranous portion of

17

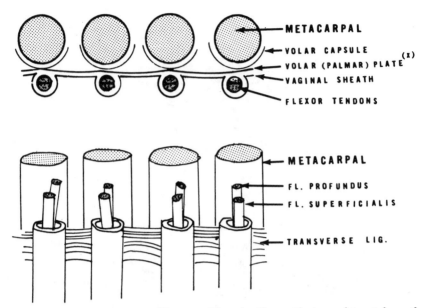

FIGURE 20. Transverse metacarpal ligament. The volar fibrocartilaginous plate reinforces the joint capsule. It also forms the dorsal portion of the vaginal ligament that forms pouches that encircle the flexor tendons as part of the tendons' gliding mechanism.

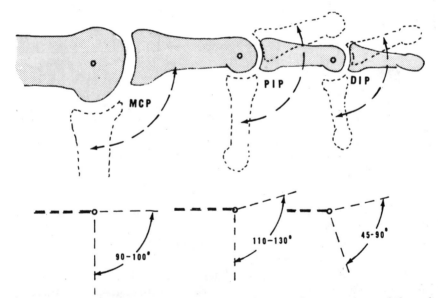

FIGURE 21. Range of motion of the interphalangeal joints. The proximal interphalangeal joint (PIP) averages 110 to 130° and the distal phalangeal joints (DIP) 45 to 90°. Both of these joints are capable of hyperextension. Further flexion is checked by the dorsal capsule. The metacarpophalangeal joint (MCP) has a range of 90 to 100°.

18

the plate, prolonged immobilization of the finger in flexion causes retraction of the membranous tissue resulting in a flexion contracture.

The palmar fibrocartilaginous plates join transversely (see Fig. 20) to form the intermetacarpal ligament. There is an outpouching of the ligament on the palmar aspect of each metacarpal which encloses the flexor tendons and forms part of the gliding apparatus of the flexor tendons. This outpouching is called the vaginal ligament.

Interphalangeal Joints

The interphalangeal joints are true hinge joints allowing only flexion and extension (Fig. 21). Metacarpophalangeal joints differ in the following respects:

1. The metacarpophalangeal joint is a ball-and-socket joint that permits abduction, adduction, and circumduction. The interphalangeal joint is a hinge joint allowing flexion and extension.
2. The articular surface configurations differ (see Fig. 2B).
3. Hyperextension, at least passively, is possible at the metacarpophalangeal joint, but not at the interphalangeal joints.
4. Collateral ligaments are tight in flexion and slack in extension at the metacarpophalangeal joints but not fully understood at the interphalangeal joints (see Fig. 18).
5. At the metacarpophalangeal joints, the palmar plates are connected to many mobile tissues (see Fig. 19)—deep transverse ligament, tendons of the interossei and the palmar aponeurosis. In the interphalangeal joints the plate is less mobile.

All these factors are implicated in the complication resulting from prolonged immobilization in an unphysiologic (extended) position with resultant "stiffness" of the joints.

MUSCULAR CONTROL

All muscular activity of the hand, wrist, and fingers can be divided into the *extrinsic* and *intrinsic* muscle groups.

Extrinsic Muscles

All forearm muscles (except the pronator teres, supinator, and brachialis) traverse the wrist joint and the metacarpophalangeal joints. The palmar group originates from the medial condyle of the humerus and is flexor in function. The dorsal group originates from the lateral condyle of the humerus and is essentially extensor in function.

19

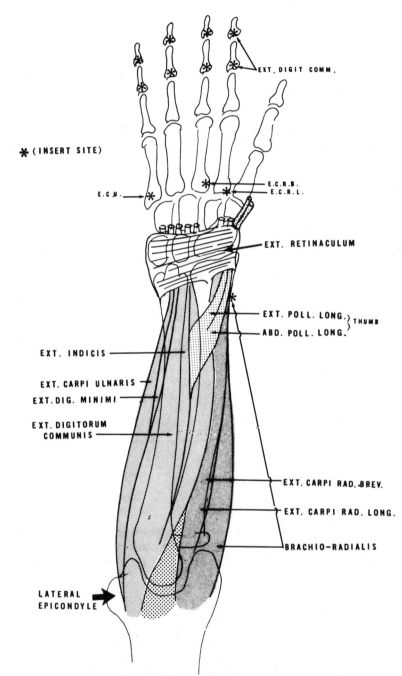

EXT. DIGIT COMM.

✱ (INSERT SITE)

E.C.U.

✱ E.C.R.B.
✱ E.C.R.L.

EXT. RETINACULUM

EXT. POLL. LONG.
ABD. POLL. LONG.
THUMB

EXT. INDICIS

EXT. CARPI ULNARIS
EXT. DIG. MINIMI

EXT. DIGITORUM
COMMUNIS

EXT. CARPI RAD. BREV.

EXT. CARPI RAD. LONG.

BRACHIO-RADIALIS

LATERAL
EPICONDYLE

FIGURE 22. Extensor muscles of the forearm. The origin and insertion of the extensor muscles are shown as viewed in the left arm and hand. The extensor groups comprise a superficial and deep layer which are divided by the extrinsic thumb muscles.

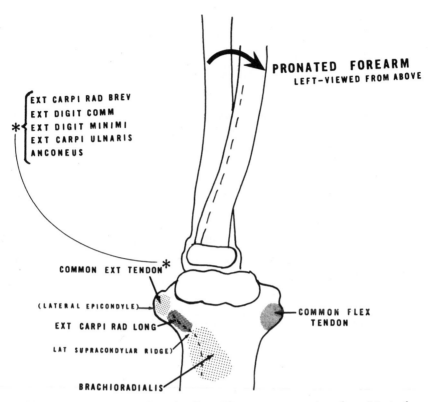

EXT CARPI RAD BREV
EXT DIGIT COMM
EXT DIGIT MINIMI
EXT CARPI ULNARIS
ANCONEUS

PRONATED FOREARM
LEFT-VIEWED FROM ABOVE

COMMON EXT TENDON

(LATERAL EPICONDYLE)

EXT CARPI RAD LONG

LAT SUPRACONDYLAR RIDGE)

BRACHIORADIALIS

COMMON FLEX
TENDON

FIGURE 23. Origin of muscles about the elbow. The common extensor tendon originates from the lateral humeral epicondyle. The view presented is the pronated left elbow seen from above.

The *extensor forearm muscles* are arranged into a superficial and a deep layer with the superficial layer divided into a lateral and a posterior group. The lateral and the posterior groups of the superficial layer are separated by the extrinsic muscles of the thumb (Fig. 22).

The superficial group originates from the common extensor tendon which is attached to the lateral epicondyle area, the intermuscular septum, and along the lateral supracondylar ridge.

I. Superficial Muscles of the Extensor Forearm
   A. Lateral Group
      1. Brachioradialis crosses the cubital fossa, inserts into the base of the styloid process of the radius (see Fig. 22), and flexes the elbow when the forearm is midway between pronation and supination. So, although it is in the extensor group, it acts as a flexor.
      2. Extensor carpi radialis longus originates from the ridge.

21

3. Extensor carpi radialis brevis originates from the common tendon. Longus and brevis cross the "snuff box" and attach to the bases of the second and third metacarpals. They are pure *wrist* muscles.

B. Posterior Group
   1. Extensor indicis (Fig. 23), extensor digitorum communis, extensor digiti minimi, and extensor carpi ulnaris originate from the common extensor tendon. Their insertion is discussed later.
   2. Anconeus attaches from the lateral epicondyle region and crosses obliquely into the posterior surface of the ulna.

II. Deep Muscles of the Extensor Forearm
   A. Supinator
   B. Abductor pollicis longus
   C. Extensor pollicis brevis and extensor pollicis longus arise from the midregion of the ulna and radius and the interosseous membrane, and proceed obliquely *over* the wrist extensors to attach to the thumb and index finger.

The flexor forearm muscles originate primarily from the medial condyle area of the humerus. This group is comprised of two categories—the *superficial* and the *deep*.

I. Superficial Group
   A. Originates as a common muscle mass from the medial epicondyle (Fig. 24).
      1. Pronator quadratus extends from the ridge of the ulna to the anterior surface of the radius, a broad band at the distal area of the forearm.
      2. Flexor carpi radialis attaches to the bases of the second and third metacarpals.
      3. Palmaris longus is absent in 15 percent of people.
      4. Flexor carpi ulnaris attaches to the pisiform and the fifth metacarpal. The ulnar nerve enters the forearm through the two heads of this muscle.

II. Deep Layer
   A. Primarily for finger flexion (Figs. 24 and 25).
      1. Sublimis originates in the medial condyle, coronoid process of the ulna, and palmar surface of the radius (see Fig. 25), and ends in four tendons inserting into the bases of the second, third, fourth, and fifth middle phalanges. The sublimis separates into a superficial portion (two tendons to the middle and ring fingers) and a deep portion (tendons to the index and little fingers). This is their arrangement as they pass under the transverse carpal ligament (Fig. 26).

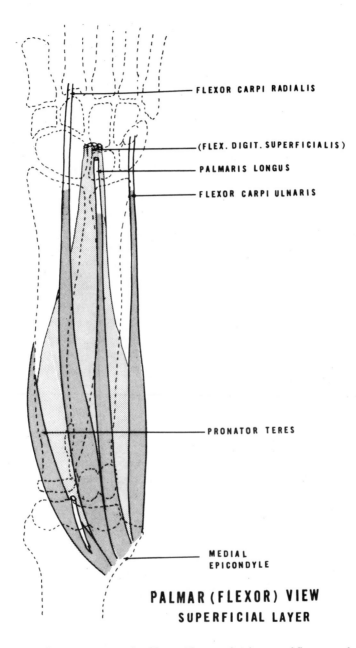

FLEXOR CARPI RADIALIS

(FLEX. DIGIT. SUPERFICIALIS)

PALMARIS LONGUS

FLEXOR CARPI ULNARIS

PRONATOR TERES

MEDIAL
EPICONDYLE

PALMAR (FLEXOR) VIEW
SUPERFICIAL LAYER

FIGURE 24. Palmar flexor group, superficial layer. The superficial group of flexor muscles on the palmar surface of the forearm originate from a common muscle mass at the medial epicondyle. The most medial is the pronator teres, then comes the flexor carpi radialis inserting into the base of the second and third metacarpals, the palmaris longus, and the flexor carpi ulnaris attaching to the pisiform. The flexor digitorum in the deeper layer is seen through the superficial layer.

23

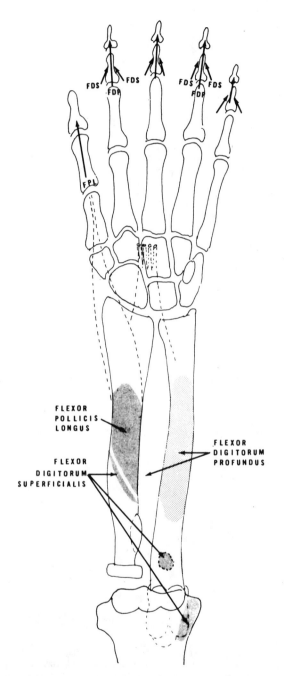

FIGURE 25. Palmar flexor group, deep layer. The deep layer contains the finger flexors. The flexor digitorum superficialis originates from the medial epicondyle, the coronoid process of the ulna, and the palmar surface of the radius. It ends in four tendons attached to the base of the middle phalanges. The flexor digitorum profundus arises from the ulna and interosseous membrane and inserts into the distal phalanges. The flexor pollicis longus originates from the palmar surface of the radius and inserts into the base of the distal phalanx of the thumb.

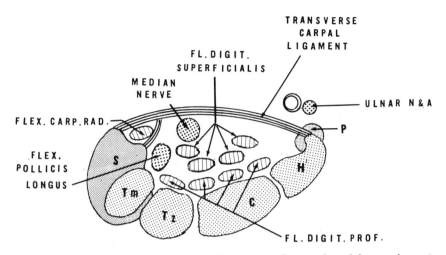

FIGURE 26. Contents of the carpal tunnel. The concave palmar surface of the carpal rows is crossed by the transverse carpal ligament. The tunnel contains the median nerve and all the flexor tendons and their sheaths. Thickening of the tendon sheaths, the carpal ligament, or deformation of the bony structure can compress the median nerve.

2. Profundus (deep) common flexors arise from the ulna and interosseous membrane (see Fig. 25), cross the wrist under the carpal ligament, and attach to the distal phalanges after perforating the sublimis (superficialis) tendons (Fig. 27).

Lampe[1] proposed a new terminology for muscles in 1951. Muscles are named by their locations, as in palmar forearm group and dorsal forearm group, and *not* by their functions. It would better serve the purpose of functional anatomy if the palmar group (see Fig. 24) (flexor carpi radialis and ulnaris, flexor digitorum sublimis and profundus, pronator teres and quadratus) were termed *flexor pronator group*. The dorsal group (see Fig. 22) (extensor carpi radialis longus and brevis, extensor digitorum communis, indicis proprius, digiti quinti proprius, extensor pollicis brevis and longus, abductor pollicis longus and supinator) would then be termed *extensor assistant supinator group* ("assistant" because the forearm supinator *assists* the biceps). Hence, the radial nerve would be termed the *extensor assistant supinator nerve;* the ulnar nerve (which supplies the interossei) would be termed *finger spreader approximator nerve;* and the median nerve (which controls the flexor pronator group except for the flexor carpi ulnaris and the ulnar half for the flexor digitorum profundus) would be termed *flexor pronator thumb-finger approximator nerve.* All these terms are admittedly unwieldly, but functionally practical.

FLEXOR TENDINOUS INSERTION INTO DIGITS. Each profundus tendon inserts into the base of the distal phalanx (Figs. 27 and 28). The profun-

25

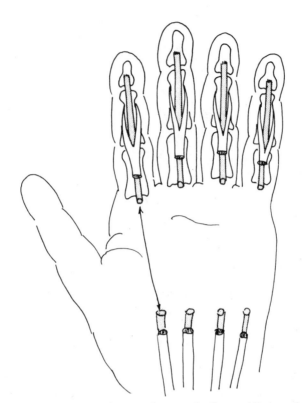

FIGURE 27. Insertion of flexor tendons. At the wrist the flexor sublimis tendons are arranged in two layers—the two inner tendons lying deep, and the two outer more superficially. In their course these tendons split to allow the profundus tendons to pass through then attach to the middle phalanges of the four medial fingers. The flexor profundus tendons at the wrist are in one layer and in the same sheath as the sublimis. They pass between the split of the sublimis tendons to attach to the base of the distal phalanges.

dus is not entirely cylindrical. When it passes through the superficialis it is flattened from side to side. Beyond that point, as it passes over the proximal interphalangeal joint, it is flattened from front to back. The superficialis tendon splits superficial to the proximal phalanx and forms a medial and lateral extension in a V-form. Each extension attaches to the lateral crest of the middle phalanx (see Fig. 28). The two (medial and lateral) extensions split at the distal end of the proximal phalanx and cross over to the opposite side. This fourth of the tendon (half of the splint) passes under the profundus tendon which has passed through the perforation of the superficialis tendons.

A tubular sheath envelops the flexor tendons (Fig. 29) containing a fluid similar to synovial fluid which acts as a lubricating fluid (Fig. 30). These sheaths prevent or diminish the friction of the moving tendon against bone prominences or at points of curvature or angulation.

26

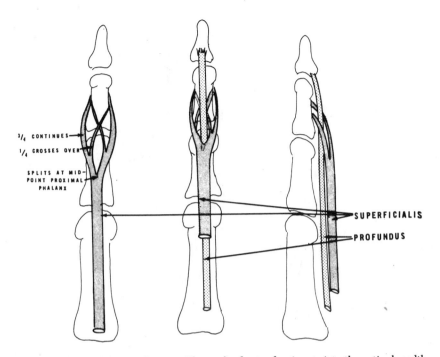

FIGURE 28. Digital flexor mechanism. The profundus tendon inserts into the entire breadth of the base of the distal phalanx, into the palmar plate, into the pulp of the finger. The superficialis tendon splits midway past the proximal phalanx. Three fourths of the fibers continue and attach to the lateral crest of the middle phalanx. One fourth crosses under the tendon of the profundus which has passed through the perforation of the superficialis tendon.

The palmar fascia (aponeurosis) crosses the palm and blends distally to participate in the fibrous compartments (tunnels) of the flexor tendon apparatus (Figs. 31 and 32). The palmaris longus tendon traverses the wrist in front of the transverse carpal ligament and in the palm divides into four bands that pass down to the four metacarpals. At the metacarpal heads, the palmar fascia blends into the deep transverse carpal ligament (see Figs. 19, 20, 31, and 32). Distal to the metacarpal heads, each pair of tendons (superficialis and profundus) becomes enclosed in a fibrous sheath (see Fig. 31). This sheath is thick and strong at the shafts of the phalanges but thin at the interphalangeal joints to permit flexibility of the fingers.

The effective length of the extrinsic finger muscles is the controlling factor in the range of combined wrist and finger movements. Neither the flexor nor the extensor muscles can allow simultaneous maximal movement of the wrist and fingers in the same direction at the same time. Thus, it is not possible to extend the wrist and the fingers together com-

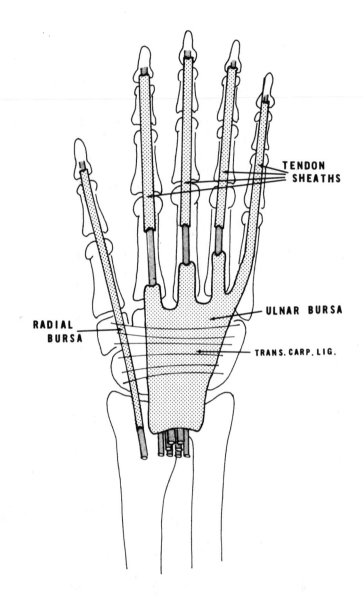

FIGURE 29. Tendon sheaths and flexor bursa. The tendon sheaths of the index, middle, and ring fingers extend from the midpalmar crease to the insertion of the flexor profundus tendon into the distal phalanx. The sheath of the fifth finger continues from the ulnar bursa which is found in the palm under the transverse carpal ligament. This bursa contains all the tendons except the thumb tendon. The ulnar bursa forms three compartments—one superficial to the sublimis tendons, one between the sublimis and profundus tendons, and one under the profundus tendons. The thumb bursa (radial bursa) extends from under the transverse carpal ligament to accompany the flexor tendon to its insertion at the distal phalanx. In 15 to 20 percent of persons, the fifth tendon sheath does not communicate with the ulnar bursa. Occasionally all tendon sheaths connect with the bursa.

28

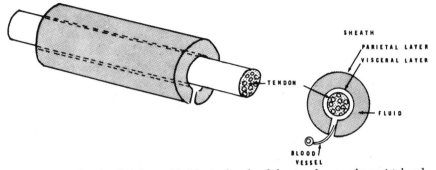

FIGURE 30. Tendon sheath (schematic). The tendon sheath has two layers—the parietal and the visceral, between which is a synovial fluid that acts as a lubricant. The blood vessel supplying the tendon enters by way of a fold in the sheath.

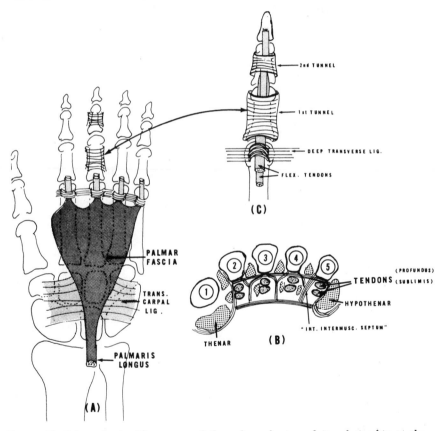

FIGURE 31. Palmar fascia. The course of the palmar fascia and its relationship to the tendons and transverse ligaments at the metacarpophalangeal joints are shown. (A) Passage of the palmar fascia over the transverse carpal ligament and fanning out to the four medial fingers. (B) The septa arising from the fascia and descending to the metacarpals to form compartments, each containing the flexor tendons and the intrinsic muscles. (C) The fibrous tunnels that enclose the flexor tendons during their passage along the phalanges.

29

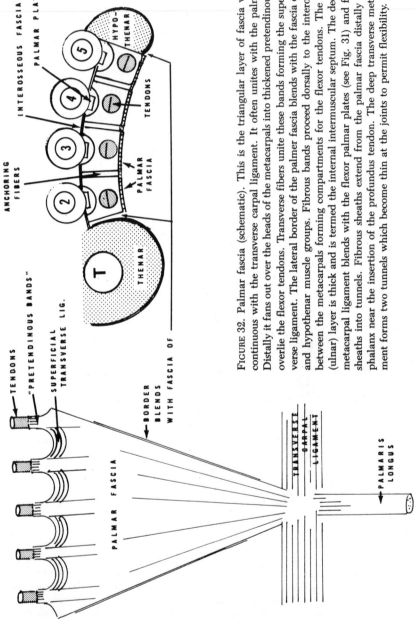

FIGURE 32. Palmar fascia (schematic). This is the triangular layer of fascia with its apex continuous with the transverse carpal ligament. It often unites with the palmaris longus. Distally it fans out over the heads of the metacarpals into thickened pretendinous bands that overlie the flexor tendons. Transverse fibers unite these bands forming the superficial transverse ligament. The lateral border of the palmer fascia blends with the fascia of the thenar and hypothenar muscle groups. Fibrous bands proceed dorsally to the interosseous fascia between the metacarpals forming compartments for the flexor tendons. The most medial (ulnar) layer is thick and is termed the internal intermuscular septum. The deep transverse metacarpal ligament blends with the flexor palmar plates (see Fig. 31) and forms fibrous sheaths into tunnels. Fibrous sheaths extend from the palmar fascia distally to the distal phalanx near the insertion of the profundus tendon. The deep transverse metacarpal ligament forms two tunnels which become thin at the joints to permit flexibility.

30

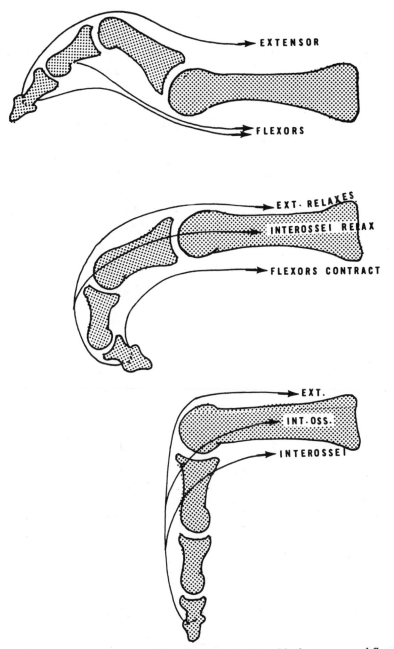

FIGURE 33. Full flexion of the digits. Normally there is action of both extensors and flexors during finger flexion. Pure action of the flexors and extensors will cause a clawing, therefore, during flexion the extensors relax their viscoelastic property as do the intrinsics (interossei). The interossei flex the metacarpophalangeal joint when the interphalangeal joints are extended.

31

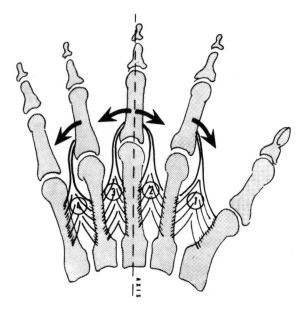

DORSAL

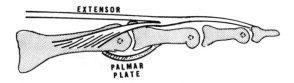

EXTENSOR

PALMAR
PLATE

FIGURE 34. Dorsal interossei muscles. The dorsal interossei muscles with the abductor pollicis to the thumb and the abductor digiti quinti spread the fingers, that is, move them away from the axial line of the hand. The interossei arise from double muscle bellies. They pass dorsally to the transverse palmar ligaments. The first interosseus usually attaches to the bone and the others to the extensor tendon expansion.

pletely. The flexor digitorum superficialis and profundus and extensor digitorum are not long enough to permit this. The most powerful finger flexion occurs with the wrist slightly extended.

Full flexion requires extensor lengthening, causing a viscoelastic action (decelerating action due to elasticity) and slow viscoelastic stretching of the interossei (Fig. 33). The interossei contract when the metacarpophalangeal joints flex with simultaneous interphalangeal extension. In full flexion there is an excursion of 4 to 6 cm of the profundus and 3 to 5 cm of the superficialis—a significant factor to consider when surgical tendon transfer is contemplated.

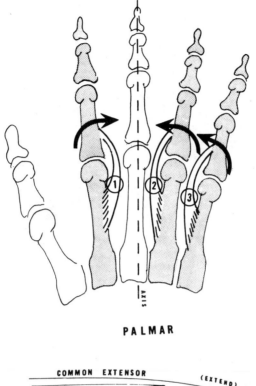

PALMAR

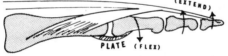

FIGURE 35. Palmar interossei, finger adductors. The thumb has its own adductor. There are only three palmar interossei arising from the second, fourth, and fifth metacarpals. The tendons pass dorsally to attach to the common extensor tendons. They adduct the fingers, flex the metacarpophalangeal joint, and extend the proximal interphalangeal joints.

Intrinsic Muscles

The intrinsic muscles originate within the hand and act upon the digits. They comprise the following groups:

1. The *thenar* group performs thumb function.
2. The *hypothenar* group performs little (fifth) finger function.
3. The *interossei* and the *lumbricals* perform abduction and adduction of the fingers and combine with the extensor tendons for finger extension.

33

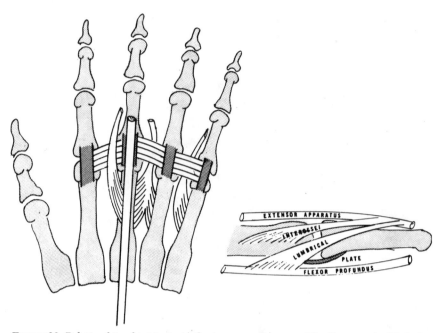

FIGURE 36. Relationship of intrinsics to the transverse ligament. The figure to the left is the palmar view of the left hand. The lumbrical originates from the flexor tendon passing dorsally to the ultimate union with the interossei into the extensor mechanism.

The interosseous and the lumbrical muscles have a similar function, though the interossei are more consistently present and stronger than the lumbricals. The interossei, supplied by the ulnar nerve, consists of four dorsal and three palmar muscles (Figs. 34 and 35).

The dorsal interossei are bipenniform muscles that arise from adjacent sides of the opposing metacarpals and converge into lateral bands that attach to the extensor mechanism (Figs. 34 to 36). The first dorsal originates from two bellies between which the radial artery passes. It inserts upon the radial side of the first metacarpal and produces *ab*duction of this metacarpal. It inserts upon bone 100 percent of the time (see Fig. 34).

The second and third interossei insert upon the middle finger and the fourth upon the ulnar side of the ring finger. The dorsal interossei *ab*duct the index and ring fingers from the midline and may move the middle finger in either a medial or lateral direction. In 50 percent of people, this muscle inserts into bone; in the other 50 percent, it inserts into the extensor mechanism. The interossei tendons pass dorsally to the transverse palmar ligament on their way to the extensor apparatus.

There are three palmar interossei and they function as *ad*ductors of the fingers towards the middle finger (see Fig. 35). The first palmar interosseus arises from the ulnar side of the second metacarpal and attaches to

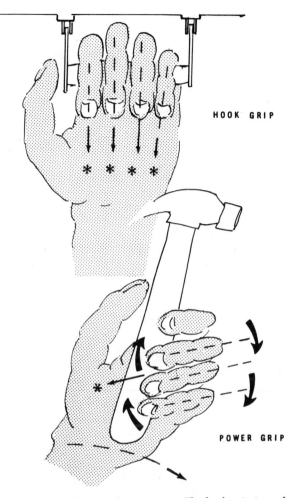

FIGURE 37. Motion of fingers in functional movements. The hook grip is used rarely but functions to hold or lift luggage or in turning a key when the thumb presses against the side of the middle phalanx on the index finger. In the power grip, used when hammering, the fingers are flexed and rotated in ulnar deviation. The fingers flex towards the thenar eminence. The wrist also moves in an ulnar deviation, placing the hammer in alignment with the forearm. The hand grips and the wrist moves the hammer.

the extensor mechanism *on the same side.* The second interosseus originates from the radial side of the fourth metacarpal and the third from the little finger to attach to the extensor mechanism on their radial side.

There are four lumbrical muscles usually, and they arise from the radial side of the tendons of the flexor digitorum profundus and pass along the same side of the corresponding finger to attach to the extensor mechanism. Whereas the seven interossei pass behind the deep transverse liga-

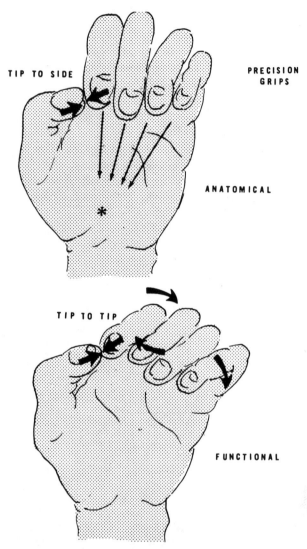

TIP TO SIDE

PRECISION GRIPS

ANATOMICAL

TIP TO TIP

FUNCTIONAL

FIGURE 38. Motion of fingers in functional movements. The precision grip requires finger tip-to-tip approximation. If pure finger flexion is used, the fingers flex towards the palm causing the thumb to first finger approximation to be tip-to-side. To cause tip-to-tip approximation, the fingers must rotate and deviate in an ulnar direction.

ment, the lumbricals, along with the digital nerves, pass in front (see Fig. 36).

If the designations *palmar* and *dorsal* were eliminated from the functional concept and the interossei were regarded as *muscles lying on each side of the finger,* their function would be better understood. Each inter-

36

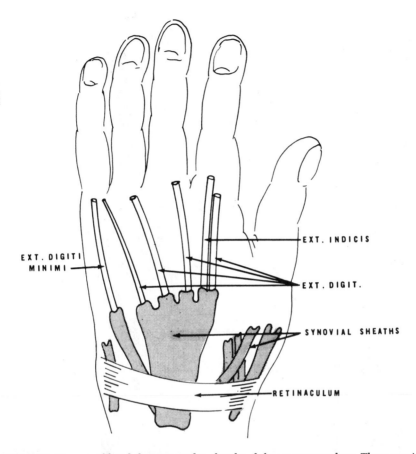

EXT. INDICIS

EXT. DIGITI MINIMI

EXT. DIGIT.

SYNOVIAL SHEATHS

RETINACULUM

FIGURE 39. Dorsum of hand showing tendon sheaths of the extensor tendons. There are six fibro-osseous tunnels (synovial sheaths) passing under the extensor retinaculum. The extensor indicis enters the common sheath to proceed to the medial aspect of the first finger, there joining the extensor tendon. The extensor digiti quinti (proprius) has its own sheath. It is the major extensor of the little finger.

osseus acts as a *flexor-rotator* of the proximal phalanx and extensor of the distal two phalanges. The first dorsal interosseus is a *flexor-radial deviator* and *rotator* of the metacarpophalangeal joint. It also extends the two distal joints of the index finger. The interossei of the other fingers *flex* and *rotate* these fingers and go predominantly to the ulnar side. They too are extensors of the distal two digits.

The lumbricals are predominantly interphalangeal extensors but they are not used for strength. They are richly innervated with sensory end organs and it is conceivable that they are most valuable in proprioceptive balance between the flexors and extensors in the precision action of the fingers. Long[2] has revealed essentially *no* lumbrical activity during power

37

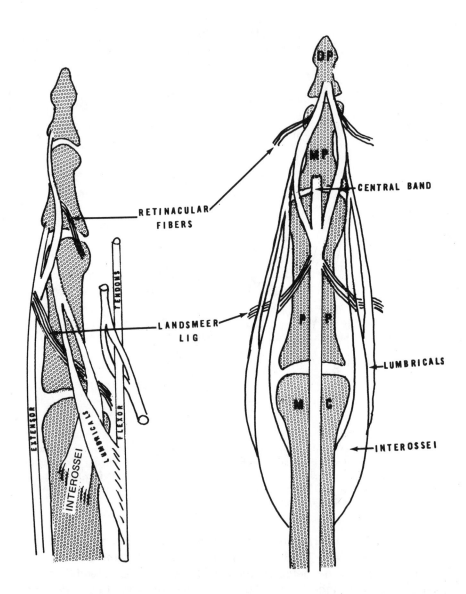

FIGURE 40. Extensor apparatus of the fingers. The extensor communis tendon divides into three components at the distal end of the proximal phalanx—a central and two lateral bands. The central band inserts into the proximal end of the middle phalanx (MP). The lateral bands pass over the lateral aspects of the proximal interphalangeal joints to converge over the middle phalanx and insert into the proximal portion of the distal phalanx (DP). A thin layer of fascia extends laterally from the extensor tendon forming a hood that encircles the interossei and lumbrical muscles (Figs. 45 and 46).

38

grip. As shown in Figure 37, a hammering position requires a firm grip in which the fingers flex in marked *ulnar* deviation and rotation to bring them into opposition with the thenar eminence. There is also ulnar deviation of the wrist to bring the hammer handle in alignment with the forearm. Wrist motion in this plane effects the action.

In precision grip, there must be tip-to-tip opposition of the thumb and finger; this requires rotation and ulnar deviation of the index finger (Fig. 38). Pure anatomic finger flexion produces thumb tip-to-index side contact. These motions utilizing rotation and ulnar deviation are proprioceptively controlled through the action of the interossei upon the proximal phalanges and the richly innervated lumbricals.

EXTENSOR DIGITAL MECHANISM. The four tendons of the extensor digitorum pass over the dorsum of the hand and under the extensor retinaculum at the wrist where they are enclosed in a synovial sheath (Fig. 39). They then proceed to the dorsum of the phalanges.

The extensor tendon splits at the distal end of the proximal phalanx and joins with the intrinsic musculature (lumbricals and interossei) to form the *extensor apparatus* of the finger (Fig. 40). Each lateral band is joined by half of an interosseous muscle tendon. More distally each is joined by the lumbrical tendon uniting on the dorsum of the proximal phalanx and attaching to the middle and distal phalanges in conjunction with the lateral bands of the extensor expansion (Fig. 41).

Without the combined action of the intrinsics, *pure* extensor digitorum action would extend the metacarpophalangeal joint and flex the interphalangeal joints. This is due to the active pull of the extensors and the passive pull of the flexor digitorum profundus (Fig. 42).

Extension of the fingers requires combined action of the long extensors and the intrinsics. Extension of the proximal interphalangeal joint occurs because of combined action of three elements. The central band of the extensor tendon (see Fig. 40) inserts into the base of the middle phalanx

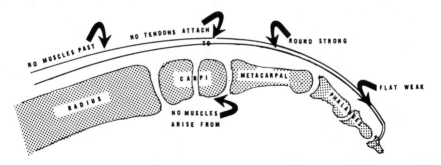

FIGURE 41. Dorsal tendon course (schematic). The course, points of attachment, and areas of attachment of the extensor tendons on the dorsum of the hand and fingers are shown.

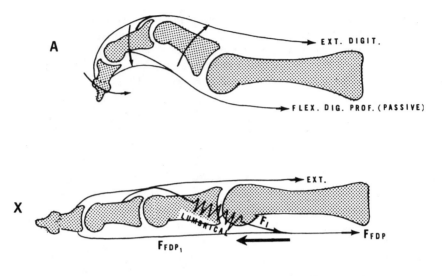

$$F_I + F_{FDP_1} = F_{FDP} \quad \therefore \ F_I = 0$$

FIGURE 42. Combined action of the long extensors and intrinsics. (A) Pure extensor tendon pull (without intrinsics) extends the metacarpophalangeal and flexes the proximal interphalangeal joints owing to *passive* pull of the flexors on the distal phalanges. (X) As the extensor contracts, the F_{fdp} (flexor) relaxes. The interossei F_1 contracts drawing the flexor tendon forward to decrease the passive pull of the flexors. $F_1 = 0$ indicates *no flexion* force at the metacarpophalangeal joint. Three muscular actions are required to extend the fingers— *(1)* extensor digitorum longus, *(2)* passive profundus, and *(3)* lumbrical pull upon the flexor tendon in a distal direction to relax the passive pull.

and the two lateral bands pass to either side of the proximal interphalangeal joint to fuse distally on the mid-dorsum of the middle phalanx to ultimately insert into the distal phalanx.

Extension of the middle phalanx is by the central slip, and the distal phalanx by the two combined slips. The length of the central and both lateral slips must be in proper alignment ("balance") to effectively extend the finger. This is why injury to or disease of these tissues creates such need for precise surgical repair. The retinacular system is *not* related to extension of the proximal joint nor, contrary to Stack's[3] concept, significantly to extension of the distal phalanx. Many authors have shown that complete extension of the interphalangeal joints can be accomplished by the long extensors or intrinsics *alone* so long as the metacarpophalangeal joint does not hyperextend.

The lateral bands migrate dorsally as the proximal interphalangeal joint extends (Figs. 43 and 44). This is permitted by the elastic quality of the triangular ligament.

At the distal end of the metacarpal, the extensor tendon flattens to resemble a fascia and wraps around the proximal phalanx forming an

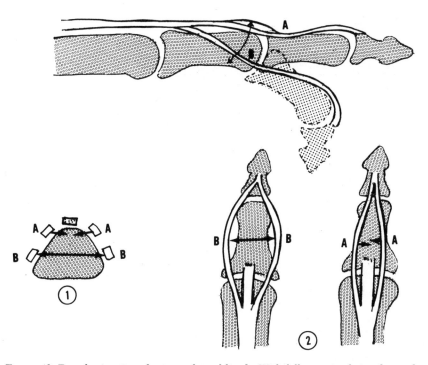

FIGURE 43. Dorsal migration of extensor lateral bands. With full extension being due to the shape of the phalanx (1), and the bands becoming taut (upper figure, A), on the dorsum the bands extend approximately from (A) to (A). In (2), the left figure is the flexed phalanx, and the right figure the extended phalanx. The lateral bands migrate dorsally as the proximal interphalangeal joint extends. This is permitted by the elastic quality of the triangular ligament.

expansion or a hood. This hood goes around the phalanx attaching to the transverse metacarpal ligament (Figs. 45 and 46).

The intrinsic muscles originate in the palmar aspect of the hand and pass to the dorsum of the extensor apparatus. They pass *palmar* to the joint fulcrum of the metacarpophalangeal joint and thus flex this joint (Fig. 47). They then pass *dorsal* to the fulcrum of the proximal and distal interphalangeal joints and extend these joints. As the proximal interphalangeal joint is brought into extension the retinacular ligament is placed under tension and extends the distal interphalangeal joints (tenodesis action) (see Fig. 44). The two joints move in concert and always at the same angle.[3] The oblique retinacular ligament extends the distal joint from 90 to 45° and the lateral bands from 45° to full extension (0°). This concept has been refuted by Harris and Rutledge,[4] who sectioned the retinacular ligament and found no loss of extension from 70 to 90°. It was their conclusion that active extension of the distal phalanx is therefore caused entirely by the lateral bands, with the retinacular ligaments acting

41

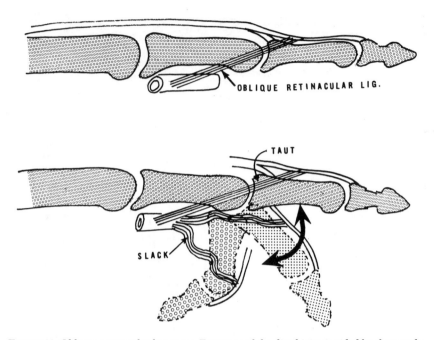

FIGURE 44. Oblique retinacular ligament. Extension of the distal joint is aided by the tenodesis action of the retinacular ligament as the proximal joint extends. In the flexed position, the ligament is slack.

as stabilizers by maintaining the central position of the extensor tendon. Hood action appears to be the most effective extensor of the proximal phalanx.

During forceful gripping, primarily a function of the *extrinsic flexor*, an unusual amount of extensor activity is noted by electromyogram. As the extensors should primarily open the grip, it is postulated that the extensor activity prevents palmar subluxation of the metacarpophalangeal joint.

The extensor tendons of the index and little fingers are joined on their medial sides at the metacarpophalangeal joints with isolated tendons—extensor indicis to the index finger and the extensor digiti minimi to the little finger. The extensor indicis enters the same fibrous tunnel as the common tendons, but the extensor digiti minimi has its own sheath. The extensor digitorum tendon to the fifth finger is often a frail slip, so the extensor digiti minimi is the main extensor of the little finger.

INTRINSIC MUSCLES OF THE THENAR AND HYPOTHENAR GROUPS. *Thenar* muscles move the thumb and include the following:

1. Abductor pollicis brevis—arises from the tubercle of the scaphoid ridge of the trapezium and the transverse carpal ligament. It inserts

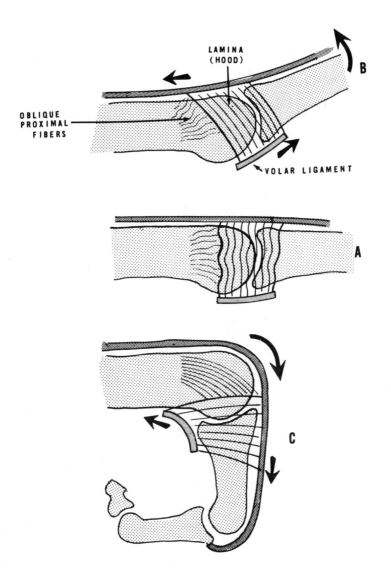

FIGURE 45. Extensor of metacarpophalangeal joint. Action of the transverse lamina (hood) upon the phalanges. (A) The finger is in neutral position. The transverse lamina is relaxed permitting the digits to be moved laterally by the interossei. In this position the collateral ligaments are also relaxed (see Fig. 18). (B) The finger is shown in hyperextended position. The extensor tendon displaces the lamina proximally. As the proximal phalanx extends, the volar ligament is moved distally. The lamina becomes taut helping to extend the proximal phalanx. The oblique proximal fibers that attach from the extensor tendon and the lamina to the metacarpal neck periosteum are slackened. (C) In full flexion the extensor tendon moves distally causing the fibers of the lamina and the oblique proximal fibers to become taut. The flexor tendon moves the volar ligament proximally. This motion stabilizes the joint and fixes the extensor tendon. The oblique fibers limit the extent of motion of the extensor tendon.

43

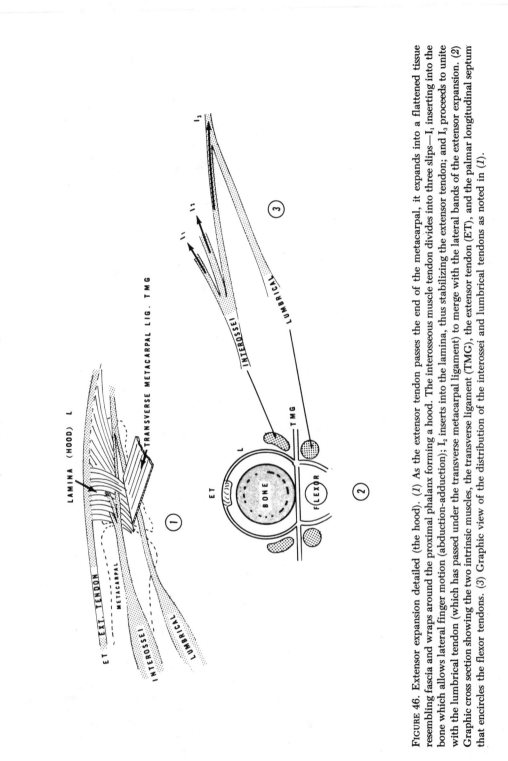

FIGURE 46. Extensor expansion detailed (the hood). (1) As the extensor tendon passes the end of the metacarpal, it expands into a flattened tissue resembling fascia and wraps around the proximal phalanx forming a hood. The interosseous muscle tendon divides into three slips—I₁ inserting into the bone which allows lateral finger motion (abduction-adduction); I₂ inserts into the lamina, thus stabilizing the extensor tendon; and I₃ proceeds to unite with the lumbrical tendon (which has passed under the transverse metacarpal ligament) to merge with the lateral bands of the extensor expansion. (2) Graphic cross section showing the two intrinsic muscles, the transverse ligament (TMG), the extensor tendon (ET), and the palmar longitudinal septum that encircles the flexor tendons. (3) Graphic view of the distribution of the interossei and lumbrical tendons as noted in (1).

44

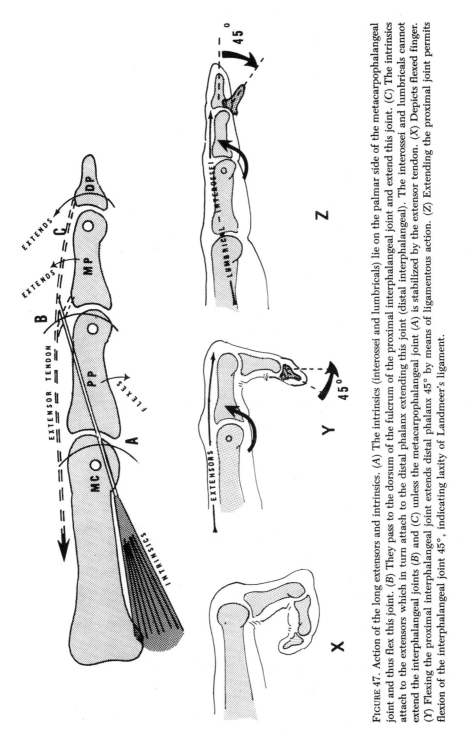

FIGURE 47. Action of the long extensors and intrinsics. (A) The intrinsics (interossei and lumbricals) lie on the palmar side of the metacarpophalangeal joint and thus flex this joint. (B) They pass to the dorsum of the fulcrum of the proximal interphalangeal joint and extend this joint. (C) The intrinsics attach to the extensors which in turn attach to the distal phalanx extending this joint (distal interphalangeal). The interossei and lumbricals cannot extend the interphalangeal joints (B) and (C) unless the metacarpophalangeal joint (A) is stabilized by the extensor tendon. (X) Depicts flexed finger. (Y) Flexing the proximal interphalangeal joint extends distal phalanx 45° by means of ligamentous action. (Z) Extending the proximal interphalangeal joint permits flexion of the interphalangeal joint 45°, indicating laxity of Landmeer's ligament.

45

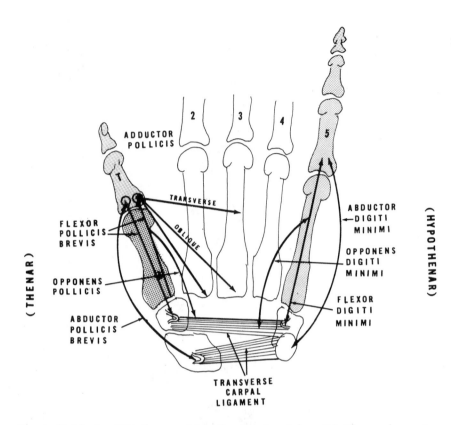

FIGURE 48. Muscles of the thenar and hypothenar regions (schematic). The muscles moving the thumb and little finger are shown. Only the intrinsic muscles are shown.

into the radial aspect of the base of the proximal phalanx of the thumb.

2. Flexor pollicis brevis—arises from the ridge of the trapezium and the transverse carpal ligament. It inserts into the radial side of the base of the proximal phalanx and sends an insertion into the extensor expansion. It has a deep portion that originates from the base of the metacarpal and inserts into the ulnar sesamoid.

3. Opponens pollicis—lies beneath the abductor pollicis brevis and flexor pollicis brevis. It arises from the ridge of the trapezium and transverse carpal ligament, and inserts along the entire margin of the first metacarpal.

4. Adductor pollicis—has a *transverse* portion that originates from the third metacarpal and inserts into the ulnar sesamoid of the thumb. Its *oblique* portion arises from the bases of the second and third metacarpals and the capitate bone. It inserts into the ulnar sesamoid.

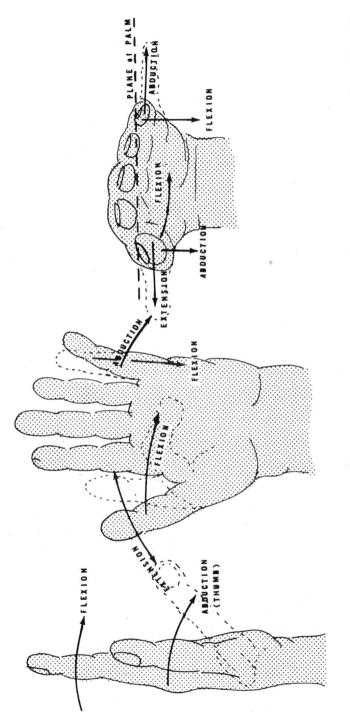

FIGURE 49. Definition of movement. Thumb: Extension consists of movement away from the radial side of the index finger in the plane of the palm. Abduction is movement away from the plane of the palm in a plane 90° to that of the plane of the palm. Flexion is made up of movement in a plane parallel to that of the palm so as to sweep the ulnar side of the thumb across the palm. Little finger: Extension involves full extension of all the joints of the little finger. Abduction consists of movement away from the ring finger in the plane of the palm. Flexion is 90° flexion of the finger at the metacarpophalangeal joints with the interphalangeal joints in extension.

47

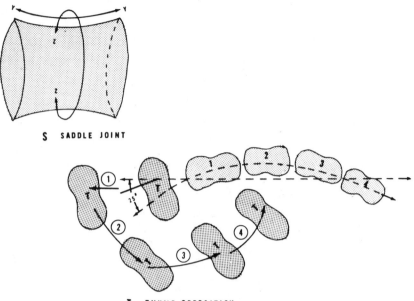

S SADDLE JOINT

T THUMB OPPOSITION

FIGURE 50. Thumb—metacarpal joint. The trapezium first metacarpal joint (thumb) is a saddle joint (S) in which two planes of motion that are tangential to each other are possible. The plane of the resting thumb (T) is 25° to the plane of the other metacarpals. Opposition of the thumb is a combination of consecutive motions: (1) extension in the plane of the palm, (2) into abduction into the palm, (3) flexion of the metacarpophalangeal joint, (4) with simultaneous adduction to the opposing finger.

Hypothenar muscles move the little finger and include the following:

1. Abductor digiti minimi—forms the ulnar convex surface of the hand. It originates from the pisiform bone and inserts into the ulnar aspect of the base of the proximal phalanx of the fifth finger (Fig. 48).
2. Flexor digiti minimi—arises from the hook of the hamate and the transverse carpal ligament. It inserts into the ulnar side of the base of the proximal phalanx of the little finger.
3. Opponens digiti minimi—lies under the abductor digiti minimi and the flexor digiti minimi. It arises from the hook of the hamate and the transverse carpal ligament. It inserts along the ulnar side of the fifth metacarpal.
4. Palmaris brevis (not shown in Fig. 48)—arises from the transverse carpal ligament. It inserts into the skin of the hand on the ulnar side.

The movements of the thumb and little finger occur in numerous planes which require definition (Fig. 49). The thumb movement is that of the metacarpal upon the saddle-shaped joint of the trapezium (Fig. 50). Opposition of the thumb is a combination of all motions; it begins as extension to abduction, proceeds into flexion, then into adduction. The muscles of the thumb which contract during firm opposition differ from those in soft opposition. Firm opposition occurs primarily from the flexor pollicis brevis.

REFERENCES

1. Lampe, E.W.: Surgical anatomy of the hand. Clin. Symp. CIBA 9(1):Jan-Feb, 1957.
2. Long, C., and Brown, M.E.: Electromyographic kinesiology of the hand: Part III: Lumbricalis and flexor digitorum profundus to the long finger. Archives of Physical Medicine 43:450, 1962.
3. Stack, H.G.: Muscle function in the fingers. J. Bone Joint Surg. 44B:899, 1962.
4. Harris, R.: Physical methods in the management of rhematoid arthritis. Med. Clin North Am. 52:707, May 1968.

BIBLIOGRAPHY

Long, C.: Intrinsic-extrinsic muscle control of the fingers. J. Bone Joint Surg. 50A(5):973, July 1968.
Lundborg, G.: The intrinsic vascularization of human peripheral nerves structural and functional aspects. J. Hand Surg. 4(1):34, Jan 1979.

CHAPTER 2

Nerve Control of the Hand

Nerve impairment probably constitutes the major disability in the hand. The hand can function adequately with a motor deficit but is practically useless as a skillful tool when loss of high-quality sensation occurs. Both proprioceptive and fine tactile sensations are necessary for skilled motor activities as well as for fine tactile discrimination.

Nerve impairment can take the forms of nerve severance and nerve compression. Knowledge of anatomic distribution is essential for correct diagnosis. Three major nerves serve the hand: the median, the ulnar, and the radial; all have both motor and sensory functions (Fig. 51).

NERVE SEVERANCE

Following an injury in which a nerve section or tendon division may have occurred, as accurate a diagnosis as possible must be made before anesthesia is administered and surgery begun. Exploratory surgery performed on a hand for nerve or tendon section must never be undertaken as an initial procedure. If there is an apparent nerve interruption but the cause and extent are not immediately known, carefully documented tests must be made and recorded. Many nerve lesions seen immediately after injury may have transient impairment, resulting from edema or a contusion, with expectation of ultimate recovery.

The examiner must establish a pattern for sensory testing that can be interpreted by subsequent examiners with similar evaluations. Initially, the patient should be asked to outline the injured area and indicate if the sensation is gone or changed. Sensory tests attempt to map the skin sensory areas. This will crudely establish gross sensation in one of the major nerves supplying the hand. Most tests evaluate response to pain, light touch, and temperature; these are considered to be protective sensations. These gross sensations do not correlate with functional loss.

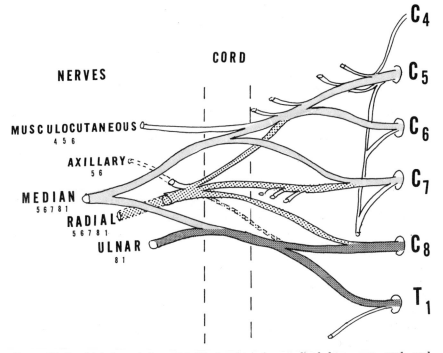

FIGURE 51. Brachial plexus (schematic). The brachial plexus is divided into roots, cords, and the five major nerves (with their root components).

Of greater functional value to the patient is the ability to localize a site of sensation with the eyes closed. The blindfolded patient is asked to identify the exact area touched by the examiner.

Testing can be with a pinprick or scratch (pain), or cotton (light touch). Testing should begin at the tips of the palmar surface of the fingers where sensation is most acute. Quantitative testing has been advocated in which numerous fibers of different stiffness (e.g., horsehair or nylon) are pressed perpendicular to the skin until they bend. With eyes closed, the patient identifies the point of pressure and specifically records the exact site.

Two-point discrimination (the Weber test) involves touching the skin with two blunt points simultaneously, with the two points placed along a longitudinal line of the finger. The patient, with eyes closed, immediately specifies whether one or two points is felt. The number is varied according to the separation. If two of three times the patient does not recognize one or two points correctly, proprioceptive impairment is implied. This two-point discrimination instrument can be made by spreading a paper clip. The normal distances on the palmar surfaces of the fingers that can

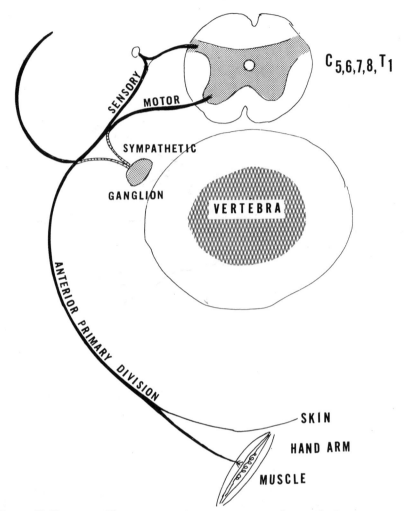

FIGURE 52. Nerve root. The nerve root—its sensory, motor, and sympathetic components—is shown as to its anterior primary division. The posterior primary division, with its branches to the skin, neck posterior muscles, and zyoapophyseal joints, is not depicted.

be discerned consist of the index finger, 2 to 4 mm; the little finger, 3 to 5 mm; and the dorsum of the hand, 6 to 12 mm.

A failure above 10 mm implies a loss of sufficient significance to impair precision hand grip. This test requires judgment on the part of the patient and therefore demands intelligence, cooperation, and patience; however, the test does not test nerve sensation primarily.

Sympathetic innervation is also specific. Only an injury to a nerve proximal to the entry of the sympathetic nerve into the peripheral nerve will fail to damage the sudomotor function of that nerve (Fig. 52). The

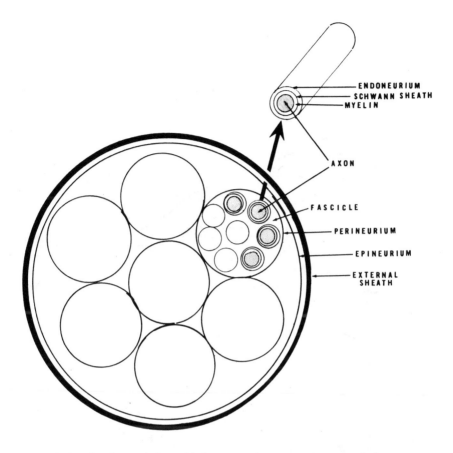

FIGURE 53. Peripheral nerve (schematic). In cross section, a nerve is composed of many axons grouped into a fascicle. Each axon is surrounded by myelin enclosed within a sheath of Schwann. This is in turn coated with endoneurium which is composed of longitudinal collagen strips. Perineurium binds the fascicles which are in turn bound together by epineurium. The entire nerve is covered by an external sheath.

denervated portion of the hand fails to perspire, and the skin feels dry. The specific loss of perspiration can be photographed by painting the hand with an alcohol solution of cobalt chloride, then causing the patient to perspire.

Immediately after denervation the hand is warm, presumably owing to paresis of the vasomotor nerves. The hand gets cold after three to four weeks.

Tactile sensory loss can best be determined by testing hand function. The patient's ability to recognize numerous small objects—such as screws, pins, tacks, or paper clips—or the texture or size of objects and the ability to manipulate these objects are practical tests of sensory function. Com-

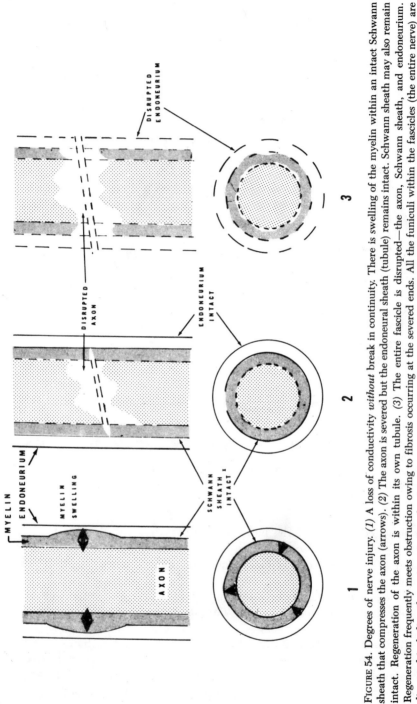

FIGURE 54. Degrees of nerve injury. *(1)* A loss of conductivity *without* break in continuity. There is swelling of the myelin within an intact Schwann sheath that compresses the axon (arrows). *(2)* The axon is severed but the endoneural sheath (tubule) remains intact. Schwann sheath may also remain intact. Regeneration of the axon is within its own tubule. *(3)* The entire fascicle is disrupted—the axon, Schwann sheath, and endoneurium. Regeneration frequently meets obstruction owing to fibrosis occurring at the severed ends. All the funiculi within the fascicles (the entire nerve) are disrupted including the perineurium and epineurium.

paring the injured and normal hands and setting a time factor for each test make them quantitative.

Voluntary muscle testing is done manually. Some form of quantitative grading must be established—from total paralysis, to contraction against resistance, to normal. Testing isolated muscle function may be difficult. It is better to test hand function such as finger flexion, thumb adduction to the index, opposition of thumb to little finger, and spreading the fingers.

The anatomy of a mixed peripheral nerve is shown in Figure 53. A mixed peripheral nerve contains fibers of different sizes having both sensory and motor functions. Fifty percent of a nerve is axon and the rest is connective tissue. The blood supply enters the nerve and branches longitudinally in both directions within the sheath. Pathology of the injured nerve depends upon the type and extent of the injury. Contusion or stretching causes swelling and hemorrhage *within* the nerve with possible residual external and internal scar formation. Laceration, whether complete or partial, causes a scar *within* the nerve that spreads longitudinally in both directions from the cut portion. The extent of the scar cannot be ascertained at the time of the injury. With complete nerve disruption, axon degeneration proceeds distally to its myoneural junction. This is known as wallerian degeneration. Some retrograde degeneration also occurs in the next one or two nodes of Ranvier.

Five degrees of nerve damage (Fig. 54) have been documented by Sunderland:[1] First-degree injury constitutes loss of conductivity of the axon *without* loss in continuity. This can result from momentary violence, prolonged compression, or petechial hemorrhage in or near the sheath. There is usually loss of motor function and tone with reduction of proprioception, but touch and pain sensation remain. Touch is affected more than pain sensation so that there is more anesthesia than analgesia. Recovery may occur within several days and is usually complete within three months.

In second-degree injury, axons are severed. Wallerian degeneration occurs, but the endoneural tubes remain intact, permitting axon regeneration within their own tubules. The effect is complete motor, sensory, and sympathetic loss within 20 hours at which point there is *no* more reaction to electrical stimulation. Muscular atrophy is usual. *Chromatolysis* occurs with central degeneration of the anterior horn cell and the posterior root of the sensory nerves. Since the root is more involved than the anterior horn cell, there is greater sensory loss and slower sensory recovery than motor loss or recovery. Because the tubule remains intact, no suture is necessary and recovery is usually complete.

Third-degree injuries disorganize the internal structure of the funiculus and interrupt both the axon and the tubule. The epineurium and perineurium may remain intact. As a result of hemorrhage within the funiculus and endoneural damage, ultimate *fibrosis* can be predicted. Recovery depends upon the obstruction met by the regenerating axon. The residual loss depends upon the site of damage—the more distal the site, the less the loss.

Fourth- through fifth-degree disruption of *all* the funiculi of the nerve trunk causes total loss of motor, sensory, and sympathetic function. Microscopically, differentiation of epineurium from perineurium is not possible. The nerve is *divided* and formation of a neuroma is common. Even good surgical approximation under optimal conditions results in limited functional recovery.

The degrees of disruption are termed as follows:

1. Axonapraxia—physiologic interruption with intact nerve and no wallerian degeneration.
2. Axonotmesis—axon disruption with degeneration but intact sheaths.
3. Neurotmesis—disruption of both axon and sheath.

During degeneration a reaction occurs within the anterior horn cell, which forms *axoplasm.* This substance stimulates regrowth distally from the proximal segment and usually begins in two to three weeks. This explains the electromyographic findings in which degeneration fibrillation occurs three weeks after injury followed later by polyphasic waves which indicate regeneration. The type and extent of nerve disruption cannot be accurately established clinically. An injury originally considered to be a physiologic interruption without discontinuity but which does not heal within four to six weeks should be explored surgically. By this time, a physiologic disruption usually shows signs of healing. Complete disruption now is evident by electromyogram. Complete nerve disruption ultimately results in muscular atrophy, fibrosis, and skin and joint changes.

Following nerve interruption, changes occur in the muscle. After six weeks, the fibers begin kinking and the striations fade. After three months, there is an increase in connective tissue, which totally replaces muscle by fibrous tissue in approximately two years. Wasting is noted about four to six weeks after occurrence of the nerve lesion; it spreads rapidly after two months and is maximal after three months. Deep tendon reflexes diminish as atrophy progresses.

Damage to the median nerve presents the greatest impairment because it supplies sensation to the major portion of the palm and first three fingers and motor function of power grip between the thumb, index, and middle fingers. Ulnar nerve damage causes a serious impairment to the person who performs finely coordinated activities such as playing the piano and typing. Damage to both the ulnar and median nerves gravely impairs total hand function and is frequently seen following lacerations at the wrist.

56

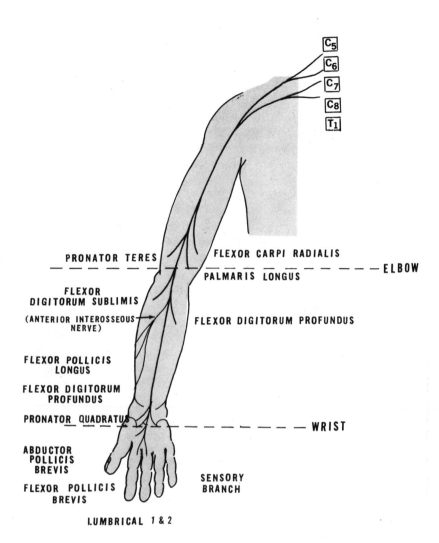

FIGURE 55. Median nerve.

With adequate examination of the hand, essential neurologic testing can be performed. Damage to or disease of the specific peripheral nerve is reflected in a careful examination of hand function. Nerve involvement of the brachial plexus can also be revealed. A specific nerve root entrapment at the cervical interforaminal level may be verified, and in a spinal cord injury (quadriplegia) the level of injury is indicated.

Currently, there are diagnostic and therapeutic measures that require knowledge of the myoneural junction of specific muscles. When electrical stimulation for testing or treatment is indicated, the exact site of stimulation must be localized with care. These sites are depicted in the figures in

57

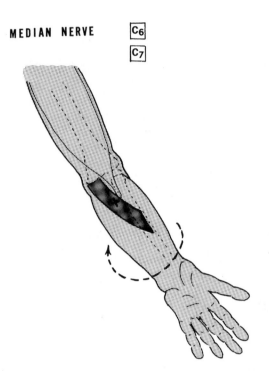

FIGURE 56. Pronator teres. The pronator teres is supplied by the median nerve of cervical roots C_6 and C_7. Its function is to pronate the forearm. "X" denotes its motor point or EMG diagnostic site. The muscle originates from the medial epicondyle of the humerus and the coronoid process of the ulna. It inserts into the midshaft of the radius.

the following sections. Electromyographic examination (EMG) is also performed by insertion of the needle at this site.

Median Nerve

The median nerve originates from roots C_6, C_7, C_8, and T_1. It descends down the inner aspect of the upper arm and enters the forearm by passing between the ulnar and humeral heads of the pronator teres where it gives off the anterior interosseous branch (Fig. 55).

In the forearm the median nerve supplies the following:

1. Pronator teres (C_6, C_7)—pronates the forearm (Fig. 56).
2. Flexor carpi radialis (C_6, C_7, C_8)—flexes the wrist in a radial direction (Fig. 57).
3. Palmaris longus—flexes the wrist (Fig. 58).

58

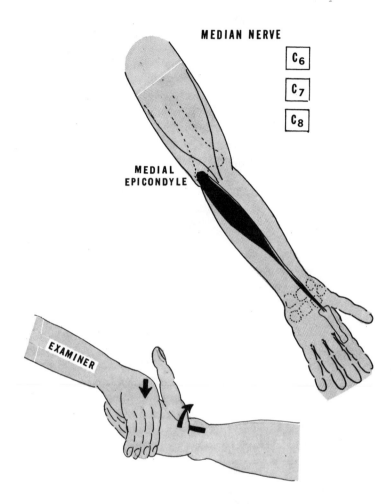

MEDIAN NERVE

C_6

C_7

C_8

MEDIAL EPICONDYLE

EXAMINER

FIGURE 57. Flexor carpi radialis. The flexor carpi radialis flexes the wrist in a radial direction. The tendon is palpable at wrist (see Fig. 15). Muscle originates from medial epicondyle of the humerus. The flexor carpi radialis is innervated by median nerve cervical roots C_6, C_7, and C_8. It inserts upon the volar surface of the base of the second metacarpal, and is best examined with the forearm supinated.

4. Flexor digitorum sublimi (C_7, C_8, T_1)—flexes the proximal interphalangeal joint (Fig. 59).

The anterior interosseous branch supplies the following:

1. Flexor pollicis longus (C_8, T_1)—flexes the distal digit of the thumb (Fig. 60).

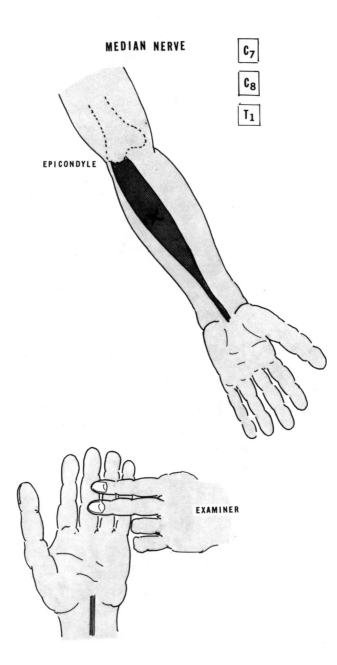

MEDIAN NERVE

C₇

C₈

T₁

EPICONDYLE

EXAMINER

FIGURE 58. Palmaris longus. This muscle is supplied by the median nerve of cervical roots C₇, C₈ and T₁. It flexes the wrist, originates from the medial epicondyle of the humerus, and inserts into the palmar aponeurosis. "X" indicates the myoneural junction. In performing an EMG, if the needle is inserted too deeply, it may reach into the flexor digitorum sublimis; if too medial, into the flexor carpi ulnaris; and too radial, into the flexor carpi radialis.

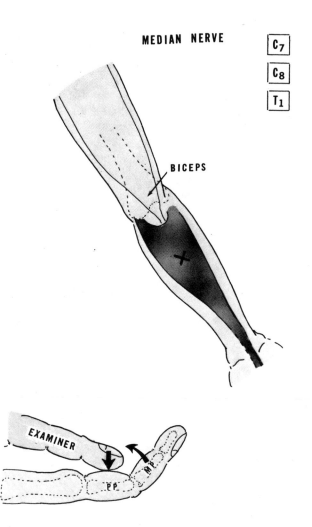

C_7

C_8

T_1

BICEPS

EXAMINER

FIGURE 59. Flexor digitorum sublimis. This muscle flexes the proximal interphalangeal joint. It is tested by maintaining the proximal phalanx neutral. It originates from the medial epicondyle and coronoid process of the ulna, and inserts upon the volar surface of the base of the second phalanx (see Fig. 28).

2. Flexor digitorum profundus (C_8, T_1)—flexes the distal phalanx of the index (second) and middle (third) phalanx (Fig. 61).
3. Pronator quadratus(C_7, C_8, T_1)—pronates the forearm (Fig. 62).

The median nerve enters the hand, passing at the wrist through the carpal tunnel under the transverse carpal ligament (Fig. 63). Upon passing under the carpal ligament, the median nerve splits into two

61

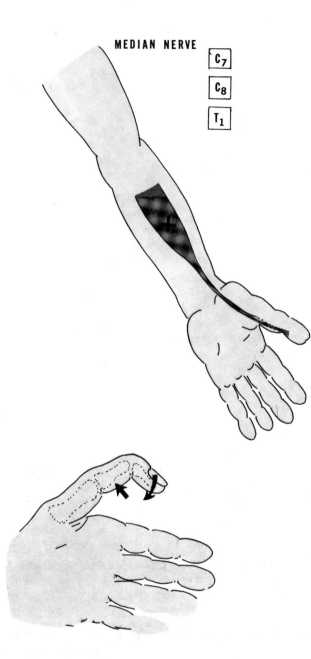

MEDIAN NERVE

C_7

C_8

T_1

FIGURE 60. Flexor pollicis longus. This muscle flexes the distal phalanx of the thumb. The flexor tendon is not palpable. The muscle originates from the volar surface of the radius and inserts to the volar surface of the base of the distal phalanx of the thumb. It is innervated by the median nerve and roots C_7, C_8, and T_1.

62

MEDIAN NERVE

$$\boxed{C_8}$$
$$\boxed{T_1}$$

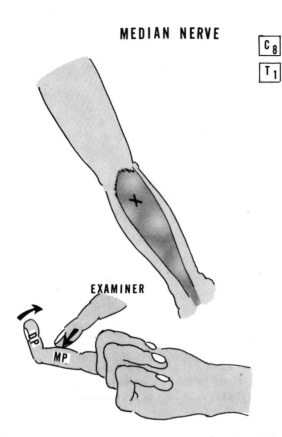

FIGURE 61. Flexor digitorum profundus. Examiner restricts the middle phalanx flexion, and the flexor digitorum profundus flexes the distal phalanx.

branches. The lateral branch is essentially motor and supplies the following:

1. Abductor pollicis brevis (C_8, T_1)—elevates the thumb at a right angle to the plane of the palm (Fig. 64).
2. Flexor pollicis brevis (C_8, T_1)—flexes the metacarpophalangeal joint at the thumb (Fig. 65).
3. Opponens pollicis (C_8, T_1)—opposes the tip of the third to the tip of the little or first finger (Fig. 66).
4. First and second lumbricals.

The median branch is sensory and passes into the second and third web spaces. It supplies sensation to the palmar area of the thumb, the first and second fingers, and usually the radial half of the third (ring) finger (see Fig. 62).

63

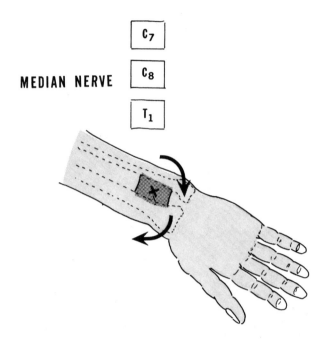

FIGURE 62. Pronator quadratus. The pronator quadratus is innervated by the median nerve (anterior interosseous nerve) roots C_7, C_8, and T_1. It originates from the lower quarter of the volar surface of the ulna and inserts into the lower quarter of the lateral volar surface of the radius; it also pronates the forearm.

The impairment that results from median nerve involvement depends on the level of injury. The most common site is at the wrist, where the nerve passes through the carpal tunnel. At this level, the nerve may be partially impaired, such as injury secondary to a Colles' fracture, tenosynovitis of the flexor tendons, rheumatoid arthritis, pregnancy, or myxoedema. Clinically, results include paresthesiae of the median nerve distribution, sensory impairment, wasting of the thenar eminence (Fig. 67), and weakness of the thumb abduction and opponens.

A complete lesion of the median nerve at the wrist results in these conditions:

1. Inability to oppose the thumb.
2. Inability to abduct the thumb.
3. Atrophy of the thenar eminence.
4. Numbness of the median nerve distribution. (A patient can make a fist, however.)

64

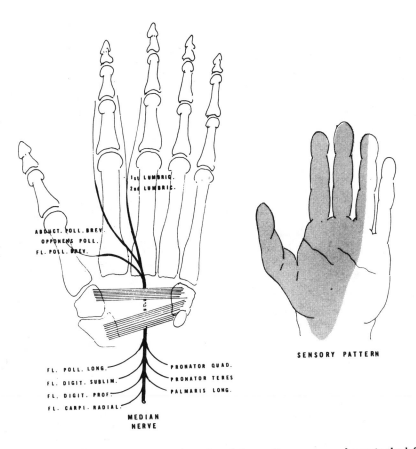

Within the figure:
1st LUMBRIC.
2nd LUMBRIC.
ABDUCT. POLL. BREV.
OPPONENS POLL.
FL. POLL. BREV.
FL. POLL. LONG.
FL. DIGIT. SUBLIM.
FL. DIGIT. PROF.
FL. CARPI. RADIAL.
PRONATOR QUAD.
PRONATOR TERES
PALMARIS LONG.
MEDIAN NERVE
SENSORY PATTERN

FIGURE 63. Median nerve. The motor branches of the median nerve are shown in the left figure; the right figure shows its sensory pattern.

If there is interruption of the median nerve above the elbow in an attempt to make a fist, only the ring and little fingers complete the flexion—but only partially (because of weakness of the flexor digitorum sublimis).

There is loss of pronation of the forearm and the wrist flexes only in an ulnar direction. The distal phalanges of the fingers do not flex but remain extended, flexing only at the middle phalangeal joint.

The level of injury can be determined clinically only by careful muscle examination. An EMG can verify the level.

In the case of a single nerve root lesion at the cervical spine (the median nerve receives segment from C_6 to C_8 and T_1 with occasionally fiber from C_5) the hand would have mostly weakness and slight sensory impairment

65

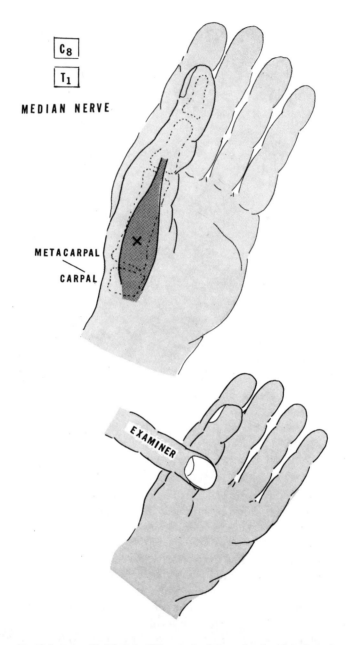

FIGURE 64. Abductor pollicis brevis. This muscle abducts the thumb in the palmar plane (see Fig. 49). It originates from the tubercle of the scaphoid and trapezium (see Fig. 48). It inserts upon the lateral base of the proximal phalanx of the thumb. This nerve is frequently used for nerve conduction tests (EMG) for carpal tunnel syndrome.

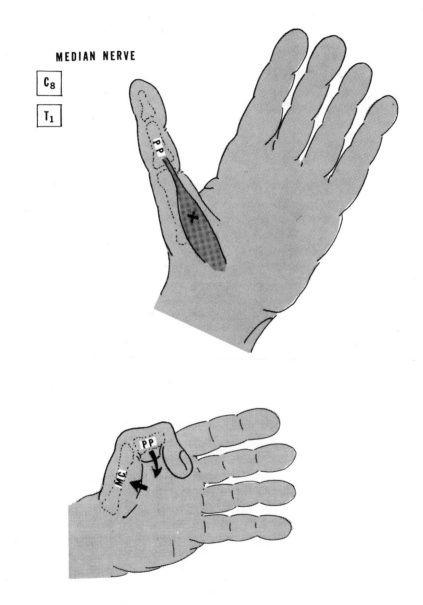

MEDIAN NERVE

C_8

T_1

FIGURE 65. Flexor pollicis brevis. The flexor pollicis brevis flexes the proximal phalanx of the thumb. It is examined by restricting flexion of the metacarpal and is innervated by median nerve cervical roots C_8 and T_1. It originates from the ridge of the trapezium and transverse carpal ligament (see Fig. 48) and inserts on the radial side of the base of the proximal phalanx.

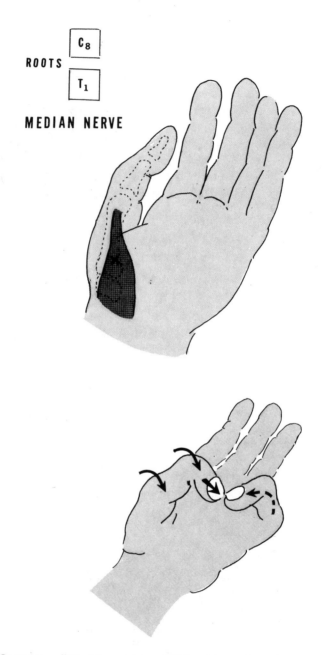

ROOTS

C_8

T_1

MEDIAN NERVE

FIGURE 66. Opponens pollicis. The opponens pollicis originates from the tubercle of the trapezium. It inserts into the lateral half of the palmar aspect of the first metacarpal and is supplied by median nerve roots C_8, T_1. It opposes the thumb tip to little finger by rotating the first metacarpal (see Figs. 50 and 51).

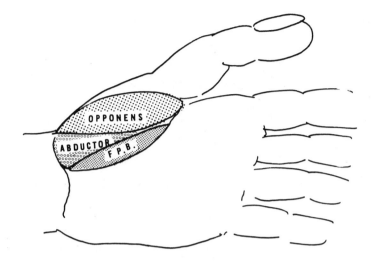

FIGURE 67. Musculature of the thenar eminence. The three muscles of the thenar eminence, innervated by the median nerve, are positioned as shown. This anatomic arrangement facilitates the insertion of EMG needles during diagnostic examination.

because most finger motions have multiple innervation. In a root lesion simulating a median nerve lesion, C_8 would be the root with greatest loss (Fig. 68). In a cord transection, the level of the lesion can be determined by examination of the arm and hand.

With a lesion at the C_6 level, the shoulders are elevated and the arm is abducted owing to paralysis of the pectorals (C_6 to C_8), latissmus dorsi (C_6 to C_8), and subscapularis (C_5 to C_7). The forearms are flexed as a result of paralysis of the triceps (C_6 to C_8), and uninhibited flexion of the deltoids, biceps, and brachioradialis. There is paralysis of the extensor carpi radialis longus because of paralysis of all muscles innervated below C_6 (see Fig. 68). The triceps may have sufficient innervation from C_6 to remain mobile. There is sensory loss of the entire hand, fingers, and much of the forearm.

With a lesion at C_7 the arm posture is as in C_6 but less pronounced. The extensor carpi radialis longus remains functional and the hand radially deviates. The pronator teres, flexor carpi radialis, flexor digitorum sublimus and profundus, and flexor pollicis longus are reduced. The biceps and radial reflexes are present, but the finger flexor reflex is exaggerated. There is sensory loss at the inner side of the forearm and the ulnar side of the hand. The median nerve sensory aspect is partially spared.

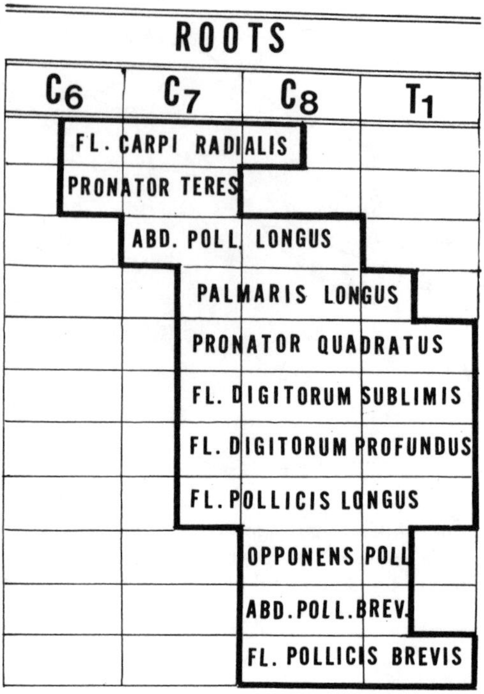

ROOTS

C6	C7	C8	T1
FL. CARPI RADIALIS	FL. CARPI RADIALIS		
PRONATOR TERES	PRONATOR TERES		
	ABD. POLL. LONGUS	ABD. POLL. LONGUS	
	PALMARIS LONGUS	PALMARIS LONGUS	
	PRONATOR QUADRATUS	PRONATOR QUADRATUS	
	FL. DIGITORUM SUBLIMIS	FL. DIGITORUM SUBLIMIS	
	FL. DIGITORUM PROFUNDUS	FL. DIGITORUM PROFUNDUS	
	FL. POLLICIS LONGUS	FL. POLLICIS LONGUS	
		OPPONENS POLL	
		ABD. POLL. BREV.	
		FL. POLLICIS BREVIS	

FIGURE 68. Cervical root component of the median nerve.

With a lesion at C_8, the upper extremeity is no longer in an abnormal posture, because the adductors and internal rotators of the shoulder are adequate to neutralize their antagonists. The triceps neutralizes the flexors. The pronator neutralizes the supinators and the extensor carpi radialis longus is neutralized by the extensor carpi radialis brevis, extensor carpi ulnaris, and flexor carpi ulnaris. The long finger flexors are stronger, as are the flexor pollicis longus and brevis, extensor pollicis longus, and abductor pollicis longus. The extensor pollicis brevis, interossei, and opponens, as well as the abductor pollicis brevis, are paralyzed. Because of the paralysis of the interossei and lumbricals and the overreaction of the extensor digitorum communis and flexor digitorum sublimus and profundus, a "claw hand" results.

With a lesion at the T_1 segment, the flexor digitorum profundus and sublimus, flexor pollicis longus and brevis, extensor pollicis longus and brevis, and abductor pollicis longus and oponens all function. There remains partial paresis of the adductor pollicis and interossei and lumbricals. Ulnar sensation loss is related to the forearm and distal portion of the upper arm, sparing the hand.

70

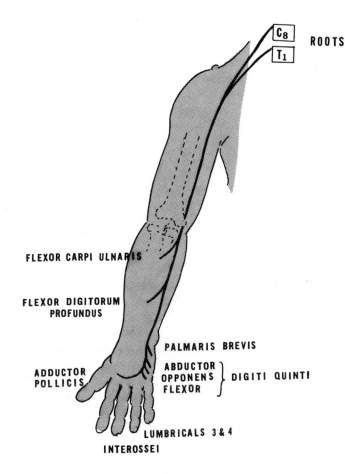

ROOTS

FLEXOR CARPI ULNARIS

FLEXOR DIGITORUM
PROFUNDUS

PALMARIS BREVIS

ADDUCTOR
POLLICIS

ABDUCTOR
OPPONENS } DIGITI QUINTI
FLEXOR

LUMBRICALS 3 & 4

INTEROSSEI

FIGURE 69. Ulnar nerve comprising roots C_8 and T_1.

Ulnar Nerve

The ulnar nerve is derived from two roots, C_8 and T_1, and is a continuation of the medial cord of the brachial plexus (Fig. 69). In the upper arm, it passes down the inner aspect of the arm, in close proximity to the brachial artery, between the biceps and triceps muscles. It passes through a groove behind the medial epicondyle of the humerus at the elbow to reach the forearm.

It descends along the ulnar aspect of the forearm and supplies the following:

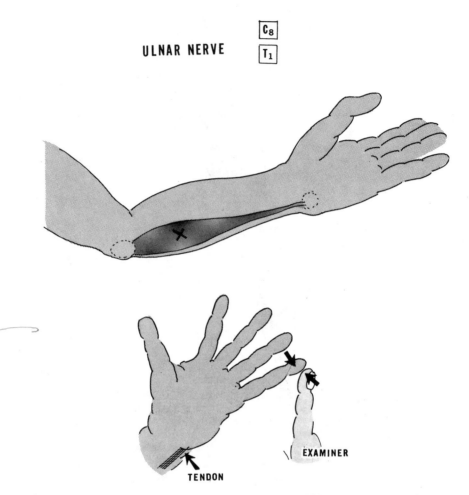

ULNAR NERVE $\boxed{C_8}$ $\boxed{T_1}$

EXAMINER

TENDON

FIGURE 70. Flexor carpi ulnaris. It originates from the medial epicondyle of the humerus, medial of olecranon, and dorsal border of the ulna. It inserts into the pisiform (see Fig. 13) and flexes the wrist in an ulnar direction. It is innervated by ulnar nerve roots C_8, T_1. The examiner resists abduction and flexion of the fifth finger, which tenses the flexor carpi ulnaris at the pisiform (see Fig. 15).

1. Flexor carpi ulnaris (C_8, T_1)—flexes the wrist in an ulnar direction. It flexes the wrist when the little finger abducts (Fig. 70).
2. Flexor digitorum profoundus (C_8, T_1)—flexes the distal digit of the little finger and usually the ring finger. The latter is often innervated by the median nerve (Fig. 71).

In the upper part of the forearm, the ulnar nerve passes between the humeral and ulnar heads of the flexor carpi ulnaris muscle. Approaching

72

C_8

T_1

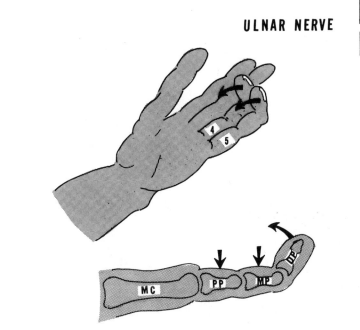

FIGURE 71. Flexor digitorum profundus. It flexes the distal phalanx and is tested by fixing the middle and proximal phalanx. It is supplied by ulnar nerve roots C_8, T_1. Muscle originates from the midulnar bone and interosseous membrane (see Fig. 25). It inserts into the base of the distal phalanx (see Fig. 28).

the wrist, it becomes superficial and lies near the ulnar artery (see Fig. 15). Near the pisiform bone (see Fig. 12), the ulnar nerve gives off a palmar branch that innervates the skin of the ulnar aspect of the hand (Fig. 72) and a dorsal branch that supplies the ulnar part of the hand (Fig. 73).

At the pisiform bone, the ulnar nerve divides into its terminal branches: the superficial terminal branch, which is sensory, and a deep terminal branch, which rounds the hamate (see Fig. 48) beneath the flexor digiti minimi and supplies the following:

1. Abductor digiti minimi (brevis)—abducts the little finger on the plane of the palm (see Fig. 49).
2. Opponens digiti minimi—opposes the little finger toward the thumb.
3. Adductor pollicis—adducts the thumb in the plane of the palm.
4. Palmar interossei—adducts the fingers toward the midline (see Fig. 35).

73

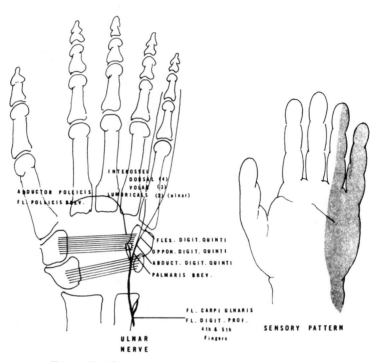

INTEROSSEI
DORSAL (4)
VOLAR (3)
LUMBRICALS (2) (ulnar)

ADDUCTOR POLLICIS
FL. POLLICIS BREV.

FLEX. DIGIT. QUINTI
OPPON. DIGIT. QUINTI
ABDUCT. DIGIT. QUINTI
PALMARIS BREV.

FL. CARPI ULNARIS
FL. DIGIT. PROF.
4th & 5th
Fingers

ULNAR
NERVE

SENSORY PATTERN

FIGURE 72. Ulnar nerve—motory and sensory distribution.

5. Dorsal interossei—abducts all the fingers away from the midline (see Fig. 34).

The lumbricals (see Figs. 34 to 36) can be tested in isolated movement by extending the interphalangeal joints with the metacarpophalangeal joint extended or by spreading or adducting the fully extended fingers.

Severance of the ulnar nerve at the elbow causes the following:

1. Flexion deformity of the fourth and fifth fingers (paralysis of the lumbrical muscles).
2. Hypothenar eminence atrophy.
3. Atrophy of the interossei.
4. Atrophy of the web between the thumb and index finger (first dorsal interosseus and adductor pollicis).

There is weakness of wrist flexion in the ulnar direction and weakness of flexion of the distal digit of the little finger. When the nerve is interrupted at the wrist, there is weakness in abducting and adducting the fingers.

Ulnar loss at the wrist causes loss of adductor sweep of the thumb. Normally, the thumb, as it adducts, sweeps across the heads of the meta-

74

ULNAR NERVE
(SENSORY)

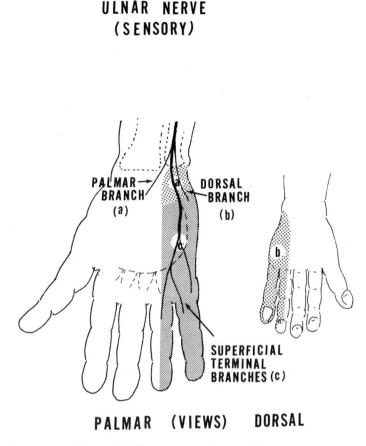

PALMAR → BRANCH
(a)

DORSAL BRANCH
(b)

SUPERFICIAL TERMINAL BRANCHES (c)

PALMAR (VIEWS) DORSAL

FIGURE 73. Ulnar nerve—sensory pattern.

carpals and maintains continuous contact with the palm. Ulnar paralysis also causes a *positive Froment's sign,* which implies the patient's inability to grasp a piece of paper between the thumb and the radial side of the palm. Abduction of the index finger in the palmar plane is lost. Care must be exercised in this determination because this motion can be mimicked by the extensor digitorum.

An innervation anomaly is possible creating an *all-ulnar hand* in which all the small muscles of the hand receive their supply from the ulnar nerve. Variations in different combinations are also possible.

In summary, the median nerve supplies opposition of the thumb to the index and middle fingers and is essential for *precision grip.* The ulnar nerve is essential for *power grip,* controling the ulnar deviation of the fingers (see Fig. 37) through the action of the interossei and hypothenar muscles and the two flexor profundi on the ulnar side. The ulnar nerve

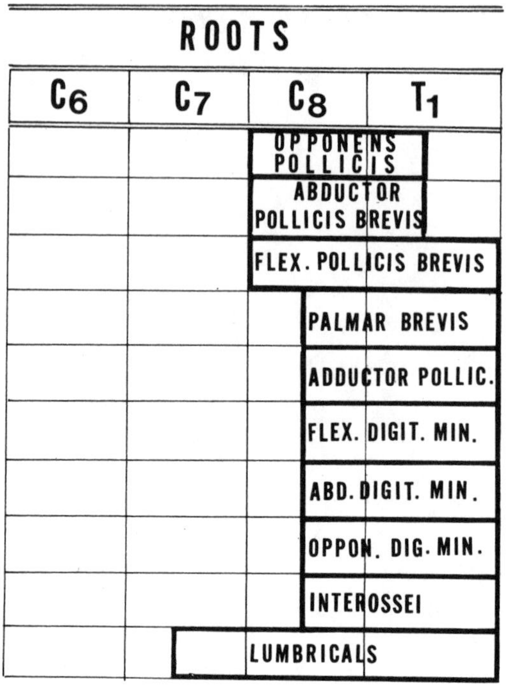

ROOTS

C$_6$	C$_7$	C$_8$	T$_1$
		OPPONENS POLLICIS	
		ABDUCTOR POLLICIS BREVIS	
		FLEX. POLLICIS BREVIS	
		PALMAR BREVIS	
		ADDUCTOR POLLIC.	
		FLEX. DIGIT. MIN.	
		ABD. DIGIT. MIN.	
		OPPON. DIG. MIN.	
		INTEROSSEI	
		LUMBRICALS	

FIGURE 74. Ulnar nerve—cervical root component.

also supplies the forceful wrist flexor (flexor carpi ulnaris). A person with an ulnar nerve palsy could perform skills requiring manual dexterity, but not heavy manual labor.

ROOT LESION C$_8$ OR T$_1$. No specific motor lesion is designated as specific for a C$_8$ or T$_1$ root lesion but any muscle innervated by C$_8$ or by T$_1$ will be weakened by such a root lesion (Fig. 74). The dermatome of C$_8$ is the little finger and the ulnar hand on both the dorsum and palmar surfaces (Fig. 75). In a T$_1$ lesion, the area of sensory impairment is in the ulnar side of the forearm from wrist to elbow (see Fig. 75). The clinical picture for a cord transection of C$_8$ was discussed under Median Nerve.

To review, there is *no* abnormal posture of the upper limbs. The shoulder, elbow, and forearm postures are neutralized, the wrist is neutral in regard to radial or ulnar deviation, and the finger flexors and thumb muscles function. The interossei and opponens are reduced or paralyzed, and the abductor pollicis minimi is totally paralyzed. As a result of the unopposed extensor digitorum communis and flexor digitorum sublimus and profundus, the hand assumes a "claw" appearance.

In a T$_1$ lesion, all hand muscles function but there is a partial paralysis of the adductor pollicis, interossei, and lumbicals, with the abductor pol-

76

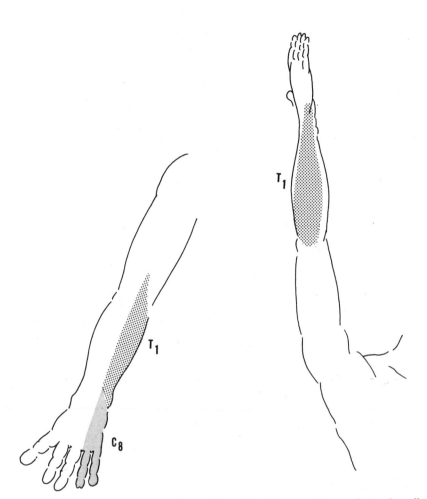

FIGURE 75. Sensory mapping of root lesions C_8 and T_1. The area of hypoesthesia clinically noted in root lesions of the eighth cervical and first thoracic is shown.

licis brevis remaining paralyzed. Sensory loss (for touch, pain, and temperature) occurs at the ulnar side of the forearm (elbow to wrist) (see Fig. 75).

Radial Nerve

The radial nerve arises from C_5 to C_8 and T_1 roots as the continuation of the posterior cord in the axilla (Fig. 76). In the upper arm, it winds around the humerus in the spiral groove passing posteriorly from the medical to the lateral aspect of the arm. It enters the forearm in front of the lateral epicondyle between the brachialis and brachioradialis muscles

77

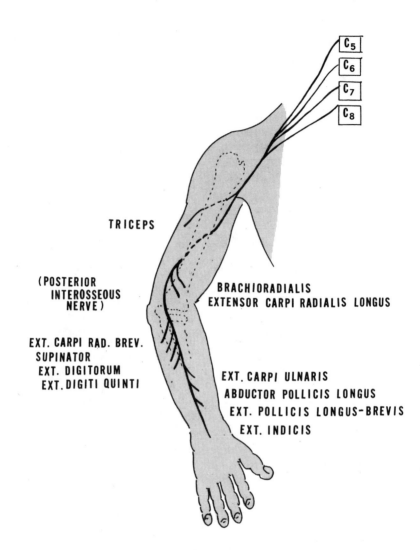

TRICEPS

(POSTERIOR
INTEROSSEOUS
NERVE)

EXT. CARPI RAD. BREV.
SUPINATOR
EXT. DIGITORUM
EXT. DIGITI QUINTI

BRACHIORADIALIS
EXTENSOR CARPI RADIALIS LONGUS

EXT. CARPI ULNARIS
ABDUCTOR POLLICIS LONGUS
EXT. POLLICIS LONGUS-BREVIS
EXT. INDICIS

FIGURE 76. Radial nerve.

which it supplies. At this point, it also supplies the extensor carpi radialis. In the upper forearm, it divides into two branches:

1. The posterior interosseous nerve (purely motor).
2. The superficial branch, a continuation of the nerve (sensory).

The posterior interosseous nerve supplies the following:

1. Supinator (C_5, C_6)—supinates the forearm (Fig. 77).

78

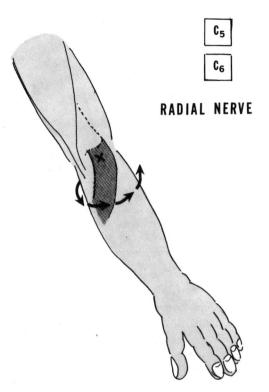

RADIAL NERVE

FIGURE 77. Supinator. The supinator is supplied by the radial nerve and roots of C_5 and C_6. It supinates the forearm, and is a deep muscle of the forearm extensor group originating from the lateral epicondyle of the humerus. The supinator inserts upon the dorsal lateral surfaces of the upper third of the radius.

2. Anconeus.
3. Extensor digitorum communis (C_7, C_8) (Fig. 78).
4. Extensor digiti quinti proprius (C_7, C_8).
5. Extensor carpi ulnaris (C_7, C_8) (Fig. 79).
6. Abductor pollicis longus (C_7, C_8) (Fig. 80).
7. Extensor pollicis longus (see Fig. 80) and brevis (C_7, C_8) (Fig. 81).

The superficial branch supplies the sensation of the dorsum of the hand (Fig. 82). A lesion of the radial nerve at the upper humerus at the lower border of the axilla will affect the triceps; at the lower humerus, the brachioradialis and the extensor carpi radialis longus are affected. A lesion superior to the midhumerus will spare the triceps.

In a complete radial nerve lesion, the hand is pronated, the elbow is flexed, and there is a wrist "drop." The fingers are moderately flexed and

79

RADIAL NERVE

$$C_7$$
$$C_8$$

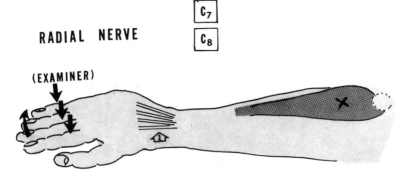

(EXAMINER)

FIGURE 78. Extensor digitorum communis (and extensor digiti quinti proprius). It originates from the lateral epicondyle of the humerus (see Fig. 22) and inserts into the proximal dorsal aspect of the middle phalanx and distal phalanx (see Fig. 40). As the examiner resists, the patient attempts to extend all four fingers (index to little: 2, 3, 4, 5).

the thumb is adducted. The patient has mobility to extend the metacarpophalangeal joints of the fingers. (The middle and distal joints can be extended, since they are supplied by the ulnar nerve.) There is inability to extend the distal joint of the thumb.

If the radial nerve is interrupted in the forearm below the elbow, the thumb and fingers cannot be extended; however, there is *no* wrist drop. Attempts to extend the wrist results in radial extension owing to remaining function of the extensor carpi radialis and loss of the extensor carpi ulnaris.

If the lesion is below the nerve to the extensor carpi radialis, the wrist extends radially but the fingers do not extend. In a lesion below (distal to) the extensor digitorum, all extensors function except the distal thumb phalanx. A lesion at the wrist merely causes sensory loss (see Fig. 81).

Nerve Severance—A Summary

The three major motor nerves are tested as follows:

1. Median—flexor carpi radialis, flexor digitorum profundus of the index, flexor pollicis longus, flexor digitorum superficialis, and abductor pollicis brevis.
2. Ulnar—flexor carpi ulnaris, flexor digitorum profundus of the little finger, abductor digiti quinti, adductor pollicis, first dorsal interosseus.
3. Radial—extensor carpi radialis, extensor digitorum communis, extensor pollicis longus, extensor indicis proprius, triceps, and brachioradialis.

RADIAL NERVE ①

POST. INTEROSSEOUS N. ② ③

C₆

C₇

C₈

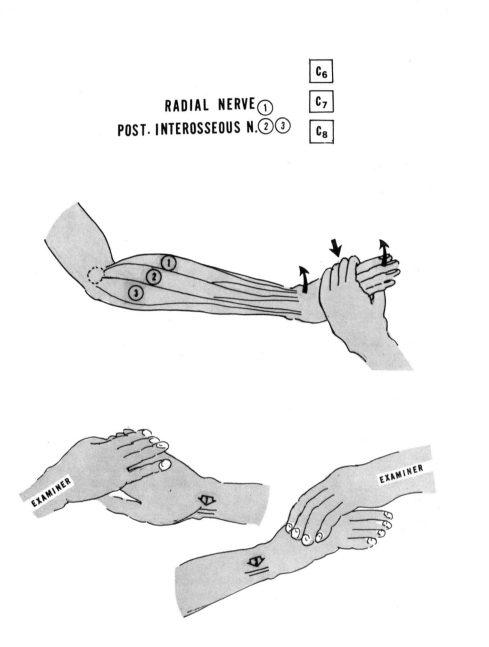

FIGURE 79. Extensor carpi radialis, extensor digitorum communis, and extensor carpi ulnaris. All these muscles originate from the epicondylar area of the humerus. (1) The extensor carpi radialis attaches with the brevis to the bases of the second and third metacarpals (see Fig. 22). They are pure wrist muscles and dorsiflex the wrist in a radial direction. (2) The extensor digitorum communis is depicted in Figure 78. (3) The extensor carpi ulnaris originates from the lateral epicondyle of the humerus and inserts upon the dorsal surface of the fifth metacarpal. It dorsiflexes the wrist in an ulnar direction.

81

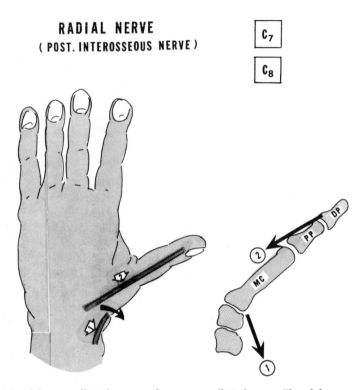

RADIAL NERVE
(POST. INTEROSSEOUS NERVE)

C_7

C_8

FIGURE 80. Abductor pollicis longus and extensor pollicis longus. The abductor pollicis longus (*1*) originates form the dorsal surface of the ulna, the radius, and the interosseous membrane. It inserts upon the latter aspect of the base of the first metacarpal. The extensor pollicis longus (*2*) originates from the middle third of the ulnar shaft (below the abductor pollicis longus) and inserts upon the dorsal aspect of the base of the terminal phalanx of the thumb. Both muscles are innervated by the posterior interosseous nerve roots C_7 and C_8.

Lesions affecting the three nerves of the hand result in the following conditions:

Severance of *median* nerve:

1. Hypesthesia of the palmar area (Fig. 83). (Anesthesia is usually complete only on the palmar and dorsal aspects of the terminal phalanges of the index and middle fingers.)
2. Weakness of the wrist flexors and pronation.
3. Inability to flex the thumb, index, and middle fingers.
4. Difficulty in opposing the tip of the thumb to the tip of the other fingers.
5. Slight hyperextension of the first and middle fingers at the metacarpophalangeal joint owing to unopposed finger extensors.

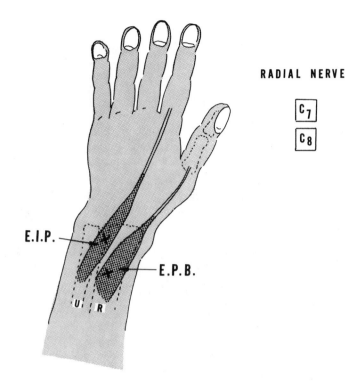

$\boxed{C_7}$

$\boxed{C_8}$

E.I.P.

E.P.B.

U · R

FIGURE 81. Extensor pollicis brevis and extensor indicis proprius. The extensor pollicis brevis (EPB) originates from the shaft of the radius and inserts upon the dorsal aspect of the first phalanx of the thumb. Its action is to abduct and extend the base of the thumb. The extensor indicis proprius (EIP) originates from the lower half of the ulna and inserts into the tendon of the extensor digitorum communis to extend the index finger. Both muscles are innervated by the radial nerve with roots C_7 and C_8.

6. Functional loss of precision grip, difficulty picking up small objects, inability to identify small objects when blindfolded, weakened power grip because of failure of thumb stabilization action.

Severance of the *ulnar* nerve:

1. Hypesthesia of the ulnar aspect of the hand (see Fig. 83).
2. Inability to flex the distal phalanges of the fourth and fifth fingers.
3. Loss of ulnar wrist flexion.
4. Inability to hold paper between the thumb and index finger.
5. Weakness in finger spreading.
6. Difficulty forming perfect letter *O* with the thumb and index finger.
7. Hypertension (30°) of the ring and little fingers at the metacarpophalangeal joints.

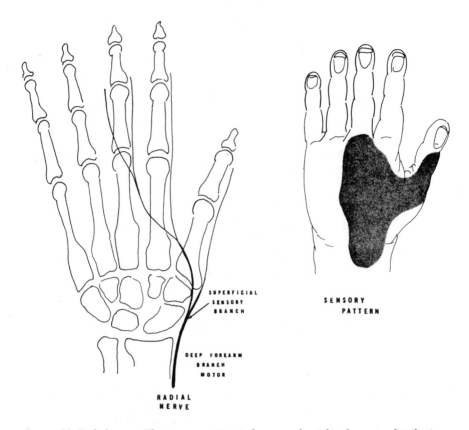

FIGURE 82. Radial nerve. The sensory pattern is shown on the right, the motor distribution on the left. Above the elbow, the nerve supplies the elbow extensor (triceps), flexion (brachioradialis), and the extensor carpi radialis. Below the elbow the nerve supplies extension of the wrist in the ulnar deviation, extension of the fingers, and extension of the distal phalanx of the thumb and index finger.

8. Functional loss of writing resulting from loss of sensation of the little finger, poor pinch grip, and loss of power grip from inability to wrap the fingers around an object; there is loss of thumb adductor.

Severance of the *radial* nerve:

1. Wrist drop.
2. Inability to extend the proximal phalanges.
3. Inabilty to extend or abduct the thumb.
4. Hypethesia of the dorsum of the hand (see Fig. 83). There may be no sensory loss.
5. Absence of the brachioradialis reflex (and possibly triceps reflex).

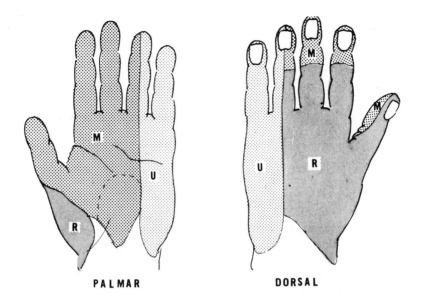

PALMAR   DORSAL

FIGURE 83. Sensory mapping of peripheral nerves. The schematic areas of sensory innervation of the median nerve (M), radial nerve (R), and ulnar (U) are shown. The dorsum of the hand is variable and the radial nerve may have *no* sensory area or merely a small area over the first dorsal interosseous.

Treatment

Although this book does not detail techniques of surgery, types of suture material, or choice of instruments certain concepts of care for injuries must be followed by any physician during an emergency. Adherence to these concepts help the patient to encounter the surgeon with a better possibility for functional recovery.

Primary suture of a divided nerve is to be discouraged and must be done *only* in the most ideal situation. A primary suture does *not* necessarily give better sensory recovery than does secondary suture done four to eight weeks after wound healing. Initially it is impossible to determine the extent of *internal* scarring expected proximally and distally to the lesion. The severed ends are usually irregular (jagged) and the epineurium too friable to permit good sutured opposition of the severed ends.

Primary suture should be considered only when these conditions occur:

1. There is a clean cut with minimal tissue damage.
2. Both nerve ends are easily located.
3. Wound edges can be easily approximated and sutured *without* tension.

4. There is no infection.
5. All proper suture material and instruments are present.
6. A competent surgeon is available.

Initial surgery of the severed nerve is for identification, close approximation, and placement of a localizing suture for later recovery and identification. Proper initial care of the injured hand should ensure ultimate recovery of maximum function. The initial treatment frequently determines the ultimate recovery, even though the final definitive treatment may be of the highest quality.

Skin closure or coverage by suture or graft is the basis of the primary care of the injured hand. This prevents infection and protects the exposed deep tissues. Closure obviously implies careful cleaning and debridement. *Care of the nerve supply takes precedence over all the deep tissues.* Surgical reconstruction or definitive repair is carried out as soon as local tissue conditions permit.

During the period of paralysis following nerve injury and during recovery of the hand following surgical repair, certain principles must be followed. The hand must be elevated constantly to prevent edema. All unaffected muscles and joints must be moved actively through their range of motion. Warm soaks may be applied locally, and the hand and fingers must be splinted in a physiologic position when not moving (Fig. 84). Materials for splinting are numerous and easily adapted.

Recovery in children is more favorable than in adults and complete recovery is possible even after a period of five years. Recovery of high-quality sensation in the sutured nerve, however, is rare.

NERVE COMPRESSION

Compression of a nerve may cause local injury and inflammation with resultant symptoms and disability. Compression may be caused by an anatomic encroachment upon the normal course of the nerve. The intensity and duration of the compression determine the amount of swelling within the sheath or damage to and degeneration of the axon and its tubule, with resultant fibrosis.

Compression neuropathy (entrapment) usually causes pain described as sharp or burning and is associated with hyperesthesia, hypesthesia, or parathesia. Nerve tenderness is usual. Characteristically, this pain occurs during rest and at night.

Median Nerve

The median nerve can be entrapped at numerous sites in its normal route down the arm from the cervical roots to its terminus. The most

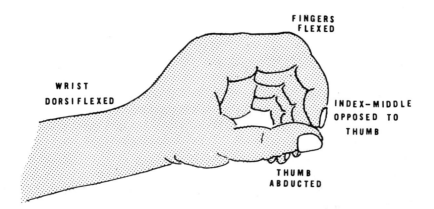

FINGERS
FLEXED

WRIST
DORSIFLEXED

INDEX–MIDDLE
OPPOSED TO
THUMB

THUMB
ABDUCTED

FIGURE 84. Functional position of the hand. This position should be sought during immobilization of the hand by splinting or bandaging. Deviation from this position is obviously permitted for specific medical reasons.

common site of compression is at the wrist under the transverse carpal ligament, where it accompanies the flexor tendons of the fingers (see Figs. 12 to 14). This is why primary suture may be difficult because the palmaris longus may be sutured to the nerve in error.

At this site the nerve supplies motor fibers to the muscles of the thumb (opponens pollicis, abductor pollicis brevis, and the first and second lumbrical muscles) and sensation to the midpalm and the palmar area of the first three-and-a-half digits (see Fig. 81) as well as the sensation of the dorsal tips of these fingers. Variations exist in which the entire hand is supplied by the median nerve, or much of the hand normally supplied by the median nerve is supplied by the ulnar.

Median nerve compression at the wrist causes motor weakness of the following:

1. Abductor pollici brevis—elevation of the thumb at a right angle to the plane of the palm. Clinical evaluation is unreliable because this movement can be mimicked by combined action of the flexor pollicis brevis (ulnar nerve) and the abductor pollicis longus (radial nerve).
2. Opponens pollicis—approximates the tip to the thumb to the tip of the little finger. This opposition can be mimicked by the flexor pollicis brevis and the adductor pollicis (both innervated by the ulnar nerve).
3. First and second lumbrical muscles—extend the fingers at the interphalangeal joint with the metacarpophalangeal joint hyperextended. This action can be substituted by the extensor communis

87

digitorum when the metacarpophalangeal joint hyperextension is eliminated.

4. Flexor pollicis brevis—has a dual innervation (median and ulnar) and thus no evaluation import.

Compression of the median nerve at the transverse carpal ligament causes numbness, burning, and ultimately tingling of the first three fingers. Symptoms are most common in women and are usually unilateral, but both hands may be affected. Symptoms usually occur during the night or early hours of the morning and awaken the patient. Relief is sought by shaking and elevating the hands, or by immersing them in hot water. Pain may ascend the arm, causing the examiner to suspect a cervical dorsal outlet syndrome or cervical radiculitis.

Diminished sensation may result in clumsiness, which may be accompanied by weakness and "dropping things." Cyanosis is noted frequently. Initially, absence of objective findings frequently suggests a diagnosis of hysteria or neurosis. Subjective complaints without physical findings may be the forerunner of multiple sclerosis but also should alert one to the possibility of radiculitis from cervical diskogenic disease, neurovascular compression of the cervical dorsal outlet syndrome, or other peripheral neuropathies.

The initial objective findings consist of impaired sensation of a pinprick over the median nerve distribution area—usually the index and middle fingers with the thumb less frequently involved. Loss of temperature, light touch, and position sense is uncommon. Slight weakness without atrophy is difficult to evaluate. Atrophy is usually noted first in the thenar eminence in the short abductor of the thumb when the condition is more severe or prolonged.

The diagnosis of *carpal tunnel syndrome* is characterized by the following:

1. A typical history of nocturnal paresthesias and characteristic painful numbness and tingling.
2. Objective sensory and motor loss on examination.
3. Reproduction of the symptoms by sustained wrist flexion or extension or by manual compression of the radial and ulnar arteries.
4. Relief of symptoms by immobilizing the wrist in a neutral position.
5. Prolongation of nerve conduction velocity on EMG studies.

It is not desirable to await objective sensory and motor deficit before instituting treatment.

The characteristic nocturnal paresthesias relieved by wearing a daytime splint on the wrist defies explanation. Reproduction of the symptoms by maintaining wrist flexion is paradoxical if pressure upon the nerve is

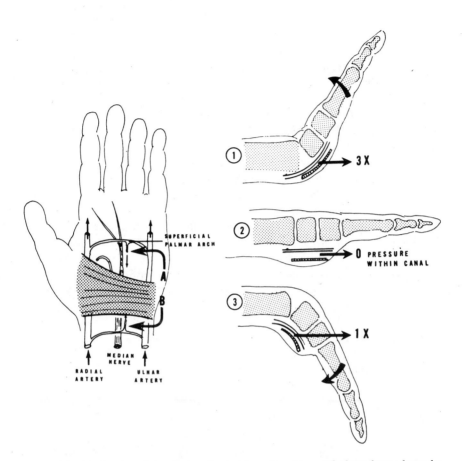

FIGURE 85. Mechanism of parethesiae of carpal tunnel syndrome. The large figure shows the arterial circulation of the median nerve receiving a small branch distally from the superficial palmar arch *(A)* and a branch proximally from the ulnar artery *(B)*. Compression can occur distally from occupational pressures on the palm and proximally from prolonged flexion or extension of the wrist with simultaneous finger flexion compressing the small proximal arterial branch. *(1)* Wrist extension (dorsiflexion), which creates three times the pressure within the carpal tunnel as is found during wrist flexion *(3)*. During relaxation *(2)* there is release of the arterial compression.

implicated because pressure within the carpal tunnel is three times greater with the wrist extended than flexed (Fig. 85).

Inflating a sphygmomanometer cuff around the arm or manually compressing the radial and ulnar artery at the wrist causes an unpleasant tingling and numbness in the fingers. Release of the pressure results in a "pins and needles" sensation lasting as long as 5 to 10 seconds. Pressure upon the median nerve at the wrist causes no dyesthesia; therefore the mechanism must be considered to be vascular.

89

It can be postulated that the nerve becomes ischemic during the day from repeated wrist dorsiflexion with simultaneous contraction of the finger flexors. This constricts the tunnel space during the day with vascular release during rest at night when the paresthesias appear. Preventing wrist motion during the day by splinting prevents compression and thus does not cause ischemia. No release phenomenon occurs at night. Space-occupying lesions—such as a Colles' fracture, Smith fracture, dislocated carpal bone, tumor, rheumatoid arthritis, and tenosynovitis of finger flexors—can compromise the tunnel space and cause nerve entrapment. Treatment requires that these be eliminated when possible.

It must always be kept in mind that the "usual" median nerve sensory distribution and motor innervation to four-and-a-half of the muscles of the hand *(opponens pollicis, abductor pollicis brevis, first and second lumbrical muscles, and the superficial head of the flexor pollicis brevis)* may vary tremendously. An *all-median nerve hand* is frequent wherein the entire hand is supplied by the median nerve with no ulnar innervation. An all-ulnar hand also occurs. Only accurate diagnosis by an EMG with percutaneous electrical stimulation can clarify these variants.

TREATMENT. The basis for treatment is suggested by the postulated mechanism. If no space-occupying lesions (such as a Colles' or Smith fracture or dislocated carpal bone) are discernible, it must be assumed there is a mechanical etiology of daytime activities requiring prolonged wrist dorsiflexion with simultaneous gripping.

Conservative treatment requires the wrist to be splinted in a neutral position throughout the day and, preferably, the night also. Merely splinting at night does *not* relieve the symptoms. If the patient's daytime activities are strenuous and cannot be minimized, and if a splint cannot be worn continually, conservative treatment will be ineffective. Under these circumstances, early surgery may be desirable. Motor impairment indicates the need for early surgery because sensory return is usual after surgical decompression, but motor return is variable and usually incomplete.

The *entire* width of the transverse carpal ligament must be surgically divided. Failure most commonly occurs when there is incomplete section of the ligament due to the surgeon's unawareness of the width of the ligament. Exposure must be extensive, but the skin incision must be as small as possible to minimize scarring. Keloid formation is common in this area. During surgery if the synovium of the finger flexors is found to be "boggy" or thickened, it should be removed.

If a patient has an occupation that requires handling tools in the palm of the hand with constant gripping and pressure, a protective pad should be worn. Injection of steroids under the carpal ligament has some diagnostic value but limited therapeutic value. Ultrasound treatment has proven diappointing. Use of oral anti-inflammatory drugs and diuretics during splinting is beneficial.

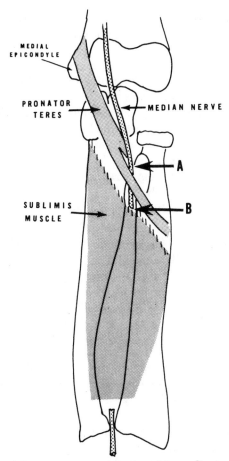

MEDIAL
EPICONDYLE

PRONATOR
TERES

MEDIAN NERVE

A

SUBLIMIS
MUSCLE

B

FIGURE 86. Median nerve compression, pronator teres. The median nerve passes between the heads of the pronator teres then passes under the edge of the flexor digitorum sublimis muscle. Pressure at *(A)* may occur due to repetitive pronation with simultaneous forceful finger flexion. The nerve can be elevated under the fibrous edge of the sublimis muscle *(B)*. Direct pressure may be exerted at the antecubital area.

PRONATOR TERES SYNDROME. The median nerve can be compressed in its passage below the elbow as it passes through the two heads of the pronator teres muscle before it goes under the proximal edge of the flexor digitorum muscle. The usual cause of compression is direct trauma, such as a direct blow or carrying a heavy object on the upper forearm. The mechanism is postulated to be a "kinking" of the nerve against the sharp edge of the sublimis muscle (Fig. 86) with the nerve being lifted and thus angulated by the ulnar half of the pronator teres.

In the forearm, the median nerve supplies the pronator teres, flexor carpi radialis, palmaris longus, and digitorum superficialis. Just distal to

91

the pronator muscle, the median nerve sends branches to the ulnar half of the flexor digitorum profundus, flexor pollicis longus, and pronator quadratus.

The muscles supplied by the median nerve along its course in the forearm can be tested clinically to determine impaired function, but confusion is possible. The pronator teres pronates the forearm, with the elbow prevented from rotation. The muscle can be palpated below the antecubital space. Substitution can be performed by the brachioradialis and long flexors of the forearm. The palmaris longus and flexor carpi radialis flex the wrist with the tendons palpable (see Fig. 15). The palmaris longus may substitute for the flexor carpi radialis.

The flexor digitorum sublimis flexes the proximal interphalangeal joints, with the wrist and metacarpophalangeal joints immobilized in a neutral position. Motion can be tested, but tendons are not palpable. The flexor digitorum profundus of the index and third fingers flexes the distal phalanx with the wrist and proximal phalanx immobilized. (The fourth and fifth flexors are innervated by the ulnar nerve.) This motion can be tested but the tendons cannot be palpated. The ulnar nerve may innervate the long (third) finger; thus the index finger is the most reliable to test. Tenodesis action by the flexor tendons can substitute both sublimis and profundus action during wrist extension, so the wrist must be immobilized in a neutral position when testing.

The flexor pollicis longus flexes the distal phalanx of the thumb. Extension of the wrist and the first metacarpal can produce, by tenodesis action, mechanical thumb flexion. The pronator quadratus is not testable.

Compression of the median nerve at this level simulates carpal tunnel syndrome. The patient may complain of burning and pain of the first three digits, possible weakness of the thumb opposition and first three finger flexors, and aggravation of the pain when pronation of the forearm with a tightly clenched fist is resisted.

Differentiation of compression at the transverse carpal ligament from compression at the forearm is suggested by the latter having sensory impairment at the thenar eminence, whereas entrapment at the wrist causes sensory impairment of the flexor surface of the thumb and the first two-and-a-half digits. Pronation of the forearm aggravates the symptoms and there is deep tenderness of the forearm. After prolonged compression, weakness of wrist pronation may be elicited.

Treatment requires rest by splinting to prevent pronation. Relief is possible by injecting the site of tenderness with steroids and procaine. When the condition fails to respond to conservative treatment, or if an impending Volkmann's contracture is the cause, surgical decompression with or without neurolysis may be necessary.

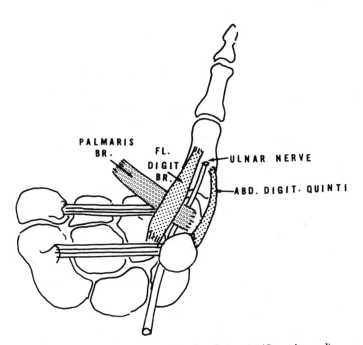

FIGURE 87. Ulnar nerve entry into hand at wrist (Guyan's canal).

Ulnar Nerve

The ulnar nerve is subjected to compression at numerous sites along its course. At the wrist the ulnar nerve enters the hand in a shallow trough between the pisiform bone and the hook of the hamate bone. The floor is a thin layer of ligament and muscle, and its roof is the volar carpal ligament and palmaris longus muscle (Fig. 87). Upon distal emergence through the tunnel, it gives off two cutaneous branches that supply sensation to the ulnar side of the palm, and the fourth and fifth fingers (see Fig. 58). The deep branch innervates the muscles of the hypothenar eminence, the third and fourth lumbricals, all the interossei, the adductor pollicis, and the deep head of the flexor pollicis brevis.

Three types of lesions can occur at the wrist: trunk, both motor and sensory; superficial, causing predominantly sensor impairment; and deep, causing only motor impairment. Usually, deep and trunk lesions occur simultaneously.

The cause is usually trauma, which may be a single acute episode or a repetitious trauma such as operating a pneumatic drill. A Colles' or Smith fracture may cause entrapment symptoms. Also gout and benign swelling (such as a ganglion) have been implicated.

93

Symptoms depend on the site of nerve entrapment. Trunk involvement causes a "burning" sensation in the sensory area of the fourth and fifth fingers. The sensation may vary from an uncomfortable numbness to severe burning. Motor weakness may be described as "clumsiness" in performing fine movements. "Pinch" strength of the thumb is noted, and atrophy of the interossei may become apparent with deepening of the interosseous grooves in the dorsum of the hand. Some thenar muscle atrophy may be noted. In deep branch involvement, pain is possible but rare. Symptoms are essentially those of weakness, especially in testing abduction and adduction of the fingers, flexion of the metacarpophalangeal joints, and adduction of the thumb. Motor weakness of the little finger is apparent.

Treatment may require merely steroid and analgesic infiltration by injection into the cubital tunnel; such practice is both diagnostic and therapeutic. When time and conservative treatment fail to alter progressive weakness, surgical decompression must be considered. The ulnar nerve may be injured or entrapped at the elbow in the cubital tunnel. If symptoms are a result of late sequelae of an injury, it is sometimes termed a "tardy ulnar palsy." Since the ulnar nerve is formed by the lower trunk of the brachial plexus (C_7 and T_1), lesions above the elbow and at the wrist must always be considered when ulnar nerve symptoms are present.

The nerve passes through a groove behind the medial epicondyle, covered by a fibrous sheath that forms the "cubital tunnel," and then enters the forearm between the two heads of the flexor carpi ulnaris. In its passage down the forearm, it supplies the flexor carpi ulnaris and flexor digitorum profundus. The wrist and hand innervations are as noted previously. Because the ulnar nerve is relatively exposed in a groove where it lies on a bony surface covered merely by thin fascia and skin, it is exposed to trauma. The floor of the tunnel is formed by the medial ligament and the medial tip of the trochlea. The roof is the arcuate ligament, which is taut at 90° of elbow flexion and slack in elbow extension. The medial ligament bulges in flexion, and the ulnar nerve thus undergoes "physiologic" compression during elbow flexion. Prolonged periods of extreme elbow flexion should thus be avoided.

With the arm abducted (as in an arm board for intravenous injections), full supination of the forearm pulls the tunnel away from pressure (Fig. 88). Pronation encourages compression. In extreme elbow flexion and external pressure damage is more probable. As depicted in Figure 88, the sensory fibers of the ulnar nerve are more superficial than its motor fibers; thus sensory symptoms are earlier and more predominant. Damage to the ulnar nerve is more probable in the case of alcoholism, diabetes, vitamin deficiencies, or malignancy.

Trauma may result from acute pressure, or repated minor pressures (produced, for example, by leaning on a hard surface or by "tethering" of

94

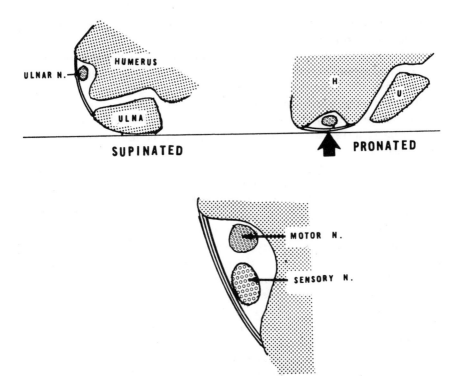

FIGURE 88. Cubital tunnel—ulnar nerve. In the supinated elbow the ulnar nerve is removed from possible compression, whereas pronation encourages pressure. The lower figure depicts the sensory component of the nerve as compared with the motor fibers.

the nerve during forceful elbow flexion when there is a malalignment of the forearm to the humerus). Occasionally the cubital fossa is shallow or the fascial covering is deficient, and the ulnar nerve "slips out."

Compression can be classified as acute, resulting from a single episode of force; subacute, resulting from external pressure over a limited period; or chronic, resulting from pressure from lesions within the canal, such as osteoarthritic changes, rheumatoid arthritis, ganglion, and soft tissue tumors.

The degree of palsy[2] is listed as Grade I, paresthesiae and minor hypesthesia; Grade II, weakness and wasting of interossei with incomplete hypesthesia; and Grade III, paralysis of the interossei and medial two lumbricals with severe wasting of the hypothenar and adductor pollicis ("clawing" of the ring and little fingers).

The patient most frequently complains of burning pain in the fourth and fifth fingers. Hyperesthesia may ultimately be replaced by numbness and weakness initially termed clumsiness. Radiation of this pain from

95

elbow entrapment has been claimed to the interscapular area, but the mechanism for this is not clear.

Weakness is noted in the intrinsic muscles (causing hyperextension of the metacarpophalangeal joints), weakness of separation (abduction) of the fingers, and weakness of flexor carpi ulnaris and flexor digitorum profundus to the fourth and fifth fingers. Atrophy may ultimately be noted in the hypothenar eminence. The presence of weakness of the flexor carpi ulnaris and flexor digitorum profundus of the fourth and fifth fingers places the lesion above (proximal to) the wrist. Electromyography can clarify this location.

Treatment of a conservative nature—such as pressure pads over the fossa, avoidance of pressure in writing postures, and avoidance of excessive flexion—has frequently been discredited in favor of early surgical transplantation. However, Payan[3] in 1970 did electrophysiologic studies that confirmed sensory recovery to be as rapid and complete following conservative treatment as surgical transposition.

Lesions more proximal, at the cervical spine and supraclavicular area (the medical cord), are reproducible by cervical motions and thoracic outlet maneuvers.

The deformity noted in a complete ulnar nerve palsy is (1) flexion deformity of the fourth and fifth fingers from lumbrical palsy, (2) interosseous atrophy, (3) flattening of the hypothenar eminence, and (4) concavity of web between the thumb and index fingers owing to atrophy of the first dorsal interosseus and the adductor pollicis.

The flexor carpi ulnaris can be tested by flexing the wrist in an ulnar direction and palpating the tendon at the wrist. More simply, it can be tested by resisting *ab*duction of the fifth finger during which the flexor carpi ulnaris synergistically fixes the wrist so that its tendon can be palpated. This action occurs even with paralysis of the abductor minimi digiti.

Checking flexor digitorum profundus function is best done at the fifth finger and involves flexion of the distal phalanx since the fourth flexor digitorum profundus is frequently innervated by the median nerve.

Tests for the opponens digiti minimi (bringing fifth finger across palmar aspect of ring finger), palmar interossei (adducting fingers against resistance), adductor pollicis (adductor sweep test—sweeping thumb across metacarpal heads), and Froment's sign (grasping a piece of paper between thumb and radial side of palm) are not clinically satisfactory. Individual function by direct palpation and visible contraction make it difficult to discern substitution.

The test for the first dorsal interosseus (ulnar nerve C_8 and T_1) is clear and easily performed by abducting the index finger. Care, however, must be exercised that the abduction motion is not performed by the extensor indicis proprius. When the fingers are in a slight degree of flexion, abduc-

96

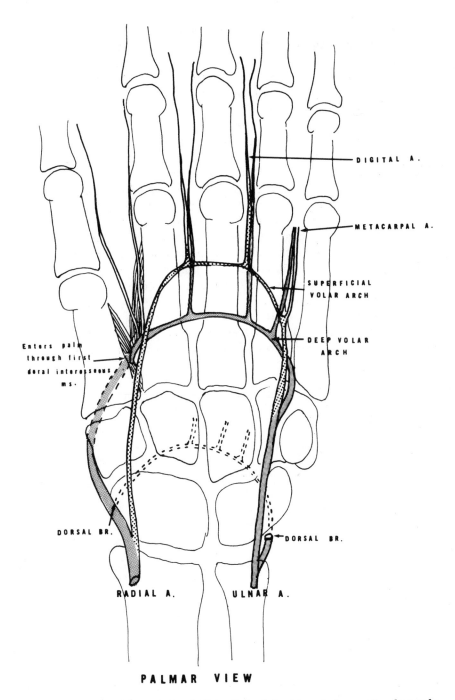

DIGITAL A.

METACARPAL A.

SUPERFICIAL VOLAR ARCH

DEEP VOLAR ARCH

Enters palm through first dorsal interosseous ms.

DORSAL BR.

DORSAL BR.

RADIAL A.

ULNAR A.

PALMAR VIEW

FIGURE 89. Arterial supply of the hand. The radial and the ulnar arteries meet in a deep and a superficial volar arch. At the wrist they both give off a dorsal branch that forms a dorsal arch.

tion can be done by the flexor digitorum profundus. To examine the first dorsal interosseus competently, proper position and motion of the finger must be assured.

BLOOD SUPPLY

The radial artery becomes superficial at the wrist, winds around the styloid process of the radius, and passes under the tendons of the abductor pollicis longus and the extensor pollicis longus and brevis. It then passes through the two heads of the first dorsal interosseous muscle to enter the palm (Fig. 89). In the palm, it crosses the metacarpals forming the deep volar arch and unites with the ulnar artery (deep branch) (see Fig. 89).

At the wrist, the radial artery gives off a superficial branch that passes over the thenar mass of muscles and runs between the palmar fascia and the flexor digitorum superficialis tendons to form the superficial volar arch. It joins the ulnar artery that has just crossed over the transverse carpal ligament. The ulnar artery divides into its deep volar branch just distal to the pisiform bone.

From the superficial arch the digital arteries arise to the index, middle, ring, and little fingers (Fig. 90). The arterial supply to the thumb and the branch to the index finger arise from the deep radial arch at its point of

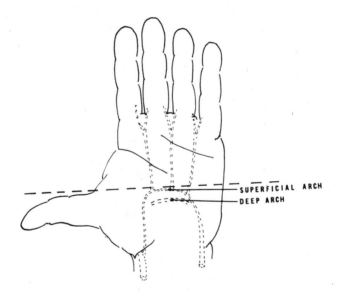

FIGURE 90. Superficial location of the palmar arterial arches. A line drawn across the palm at the distal level border of the fully extended thumb marks the site of the superficial arterial palmar arch. The deep arch is one finger breadth proximal to the superficial arch.

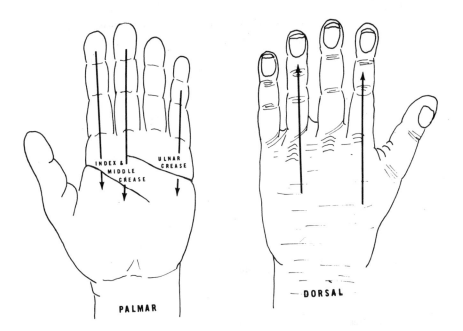

FIGURE 91. Skin creases. Creases allow the skin to fold during flexion and to extend during finger and wrist extension. The distal medial crease folds when the ulnar half of the hand flexes. The radial proximal crease folds during flexion of the middle and index fingers. The creases of the digits are attached to the tendon sheaths and permit flexion. All creases on the dorsum of the hand lie 90° to the line of pull to permit extension during the making of a fist. The loose skin is attached near the finger nail at the distal phalanx.

emergence through the first dorsal interosseous muscle. The metacarpal arteries originate from the deep volar arch. The dorsum of the hand is supplied by an arch formed by union of the dorsal branch of the radial and the ulnar arteries.

SKIN

One quarter of all Pacinian nerve endings (touch sensations) are found in the skin of the hand. When incicions and repairs of injuries are made, this must be taken into consideration and the detrimental effect of suturing without attention to normal creases must be realized.

Palmar creases occur during flexion of the fingers and are connected to underlying skeletal components by fascial connections. Incision in the palm should be made *parallel to but not in the creases*. The palmar skin of the digits is normally attached directly to the tendon sheaths to prevent

99

bunching during flexion of the fingers. The skin of the dorsum of the hand is loose and wrinkled to allow elongation and free movement during finger flexion. The dorsal wrinkles are thus at right angles to the line of pull (Fig. 91).

REFERENCES

1. Sunderland, S.: Nerve and Nerve Injuries. Livingstone, Edinburgh, 1968.
2. McGowan, A. J.: The results of transposition of the ulnar nerve for traumatic ulnar neuritis. J. Bone Joint Surg. 32B(3):293, 1950.
3. Payan, J.: Electrophysiological Localization of Ulnar Nerve Lesions. J. Neurol. Neurosurg. Psychiatry 32:208, 1969.

BIBLIOGRAPHY

Backhouse, K. M.: Functional anatomy of the hand. Physiotherapy 54:114, 1968.

Barnett, C. H., Davies, D. V., and MacConaill, M. A.: Synovial Joints: Their Structure and Mechanics. Charles C Thomas, Springfield, Ill., 1961.

Bhala, R. P. and Goodgold, J.: Motor conduction in the deep palmar branch of the ulnar nerve. Archives of Physical Medicine 49:460, 1968.

Bradley, K. C. and Sunderland, S.: The range of movement at the wrist joint. Anat. Rec. 116:139, 1953.

Brown, H. A.: Treatment of peripheral nerve injuries. Rev. Surg. 24:1, 1967.

Byrne, J. J.: The Hand: Its Anatomy and Diseases. Charles C Thomas, Springfield, Ill., 1959.

Carpendale, M. T.: The localization of ulnar nerve compression in the hand and arm: An improved method of electroneuromyography. Archives of Physical Medicine 47:325, 1966.

Flatt, A. E.: The Care of Minor Hand Injuries, ed. 2. C. V. Mosby, St. Louis, 1963.

Forrest, W. J. and Basmajian, J. W.: Function of human thenar and hypothenar muscles. An electromyographic study of twenty-five hands. J. Bone Joint Surg. 47-A:1585, 1965.

Grant, J. C. Boileau: A Method of Anatomy, ed. 5. Williams & Wilkins, Baltimore, 1952.

Haymaker, W. and Woodhall, B.: Peripheral Nerve Injuries: Principles of Diagnosis. W. B. Saunders, Philadelphia, 1953.

Hollinghead, W. H.: Functional Anatomy of the Limbs and Back. W. B. Saunders, Philadelphia, 1952.

Hulten, O.: Uber anatomische Variationen der Handgelenkknochen. Acta Radiol. 9:155, 1928.

Kaplan, E. B.: Functional and Surgical Anatomy of the Hand, ed. 1. J. B. Lippincott, Philadelphia, 1953.

Kendall, D.: Aetiology, diagnosis, and treatment of paraesthesiae in the hands. Br. Med. J. 2:1633, 1960.

Kopell, H. P. and Thompson, W. A. L.: Peripheral Entrapment Neuropathies. Williams & Wilkins, Baltimore, 1963.

Kuczynski, K.: The proximal interphalangeal joint. J. Bone Joint Surg. 50-B:656, 1968.

Lampe, E. W.: Surgical anatomy of the hand. Clin. Symp. CIBA 9(1):Jan.-Feb., 1957.

Long, C.: Highland View Hospital Report, Nov. 1968, III., No. 1. Ampersand Research Group Medical Engineering, Cleveland, Ohio.

Marinacci, A. A.: Comparative value of measurement of nerve conduction velocity and electromyography in the diagnosis of carpal tunnel syndrome. Archives of Physical Medicine 45:548, 1964.

100

Marinacci, A. A. and Von Hagen, R. O.: Misleading all median hand. Arch. Neurol. 12:80, 1965.

Marinacci, A. A.: Applied Electromyography. Lea & Febiger, Philadelphia, 1968.

Moberg, Erik: Emergency Surgery of the Hand. E. & S. Livingstone, London, 1967.

Murphy, A. F. and Stark, H. H.: Closed dislocation of the metacarpophalangeal joint of the index finger. J. Bone Joint Surg. 49-A:1579, 1967.

Napier, J.: The prehensile movements of the human hand. J. Bone Joint Surg. 38-B:902, 1956.

Oester, Y. T. and Mayer, J. H.: Motor Examination of the Peripheral Nerve Injuries. Charles C Thomas, Springfield, Ill., 1960.

Omer, G. E.: Evaluation and reconstruction of the forearm and hand after acute traumatic peripheral nerve injuries. J. Bone Joint Surg. 50:1454, 1968.

Papathanassiou, B. T.: Variants of the motor branch of the median nerve in the hand. J. Bone Joint Surg. 50-B:156, 1968.

Steindler, A.: Mechanics of muscular contractures in wrist and fingers. J. Bone Joint Surg. 14:1, 1932.

Trueta, J.: Studies of the Development and Decay of the Human Frame. W. B. Saunders, Philadelphia, 1968.

Verdan, C. E.: Half a century of flexor tendon surgery. J. Bone Joint Surg. 54-A:472, 1972.

Watson–Jones, R.: Leri's pleonosteosis, carpal tunnel compression of the median nerves and Morton's metatarsalgia. J. Bone Joint Surg. 31:560, 1949.

Watson–Jones, R.: Foreword to ed. 2. The Care of Minor Hand Injuries, A. E. Flatt. C. V. Mosby, St. Louis, 1963.

Zancolli, E.: Structural and Dynamic Bases of Hand Surgery. J. B. Lippincott, Philadelphia, 1968.

CHAPTER 3

Reflex Sympathetic Dystrophy

Reflex sympathetic dystrophy has been differentiated into *major* and *minor* classifications. The *major* category includes causalgia, "phantom" pain, and thalamic syndrome. The *minor* classification comprises the shoulder-hand-finger syndromes, including postfracture, posthemiparesis, postmyocardial infarction, postcasting, post-trauma, and postinjection. In essence, any shoulder-hand-finger syndrome of classic description, but secondary to or attributed to the numerous, considered contributory causes is considered a minor dystrophy.

All the dystrophies have a vasomotor spastic vascular component with sudomotor autonomic hyperactivity. Homans'[1] originated the term *minor*, in which he attributed a vascular mechanism to the causation of pain with resultant osteoporosis and reflex dystrophic soft tissue changes. Volkmann described a painful post-traumatic rarefaction of bone. Sudeck described a similar syndrome but included edema, coldness, and cyanosis along with the presence of pain.

CAUSALGIA

Causalgia is now considered a *major* reflex sympathetic dystrophy. It was initially described by Mitchell[2] as a "burning pain" in the sensory distribution of a nerve near a penetrating missile wound. The term is derived from *kausos* (heat) and *algo* (pain), and is usually described by patients as a burning sensation.

Causalgia is characterized by a constant, deep, diffuse, intense pain and hypersensitivity. Women seem to be more frequently afflicted than men, but this point is not universally accepted. Pain is intensified by exposure to cold, heat, to moving air currents, or light touching. The patient prohibits any passive movement of the part and avoids any active movement. The facial expression usually depicts the subjective severity of the pain. The affected part is frequently kept wrapped in moist, loose dressings and is held elevated and away from any possible contact.

The pain may begin immediately after an injury such as cortex fracture, sprain, penetrating wound, or minor nerve injury. Not infrequently, a delay of weeks may follow a minor injury before the patient alleges having severe pain. Severe pain may be claimed even in the absence of any objective findings.

The extremity involved may show vasospasm or vasodilatation, with dilatation noted first. The hand is pink, warm, and dry. The condition may then progress to vasospasm (constriction), with the hand becoming cold, bluish, and moist. Progression ultimately causes the skin to become glossy (shiny), the intrinsic muscle to undergo atrophy, and the joints to stiffen. Fortunately, most cases of causalgia terminate or are aborted therapeutically before the final stages are reached.

Although the mechanism of causalgia remains obscure, the sympathetic system is obviously involved. *Pain is the primary causative factor*, with all other tissue changes being secondary. The susceptible patient usually has a low pain threshold and emotional lability. An injury causes infiltration of exudate into the tissues, this exudate cannot be removed, since the patient avoids any movement. *Inactivity* (immobility) becomes the secondary causative factor. Further venous congestion and lymphatic stasis result in ultimate organization of the protein-rich exudate. Fibrosis, chronic edema, and osteoporosis result. The cycle is self-perpetuating as long as the pain that causes the inactivity persists.

The causes of causalgia are as numerous as the varieties of this syndrome. The syndrome has been termed Sudeck's atrophy, causalgia (minor or major), post-traumatic osteoporosis, postmyocardial infarction, painful shoulder, swollen atrophic hand associated with cervical radiculitis, shoulder-hand-syndrome of hemiplegia, and so forth. The syndrome displays varying degrees of reflex physiologic reaction, both vasomotor and sudomotor, to an inciting internal or external noxious agent.

Treatment

Treatment consists essentially of interrupting the causative cycle and must be initiated early and energetically. Although it is estimated that approximately 60 percent of all patients make a spontaneous recovery, the rapidity and completeness of recovery are influenced by the efficacy of the treatment.

Prevention is the treatment of choice. In any injury to an extremity, immobilization must be exact and comfortable, with the proximal and distal joints left free and their movements encouraged. The part must be elevated to prevent venous congestion and dependent edema. Pain must be controlled by appropriate medication. Aspirin has analgesic as well as

103

other benefits not fully understood, and must be administered in large and periodic doses, taken on a full stomach, and used with antacid medicine to prevent gastric irritation. A stronger analgesic may be necessary. "Trigger areas" when found can be infiltrated with a local anesthetic or sprayed with ethyl chloride. A painful scar or neuroma may need surgical removal; however, if surgery is once attempted unsuccessfully, it *must not be repeated.*

Perineural infusion of the trigger area has recently been advocated. The localized area is prepared for surgery, and a large-bore needle is inserted into the area until the symptoms are reproduced. Then a flexible venous catheter is inserted through the needle, and 0.5 ml of 0.5 percent lidocaine is infiltrated. If the symptoms are relieved, the needle is removed, the venous catheter remains inserted, and repeated injections of lidocaine every 3 to 4 hours for two to three weeks are administered.

Selective large-nerve electrical stimulation proximal to the lesion is applied. A 0.1 msec unidirectional square wave (100 Hz voltage) is applied for 2 to 3 minutes, giving relief for 2 to 12 hours, during which time active physical therapy can be administered.

There have been encouraging reports of marked benefit in using chlorpromazine (Thorazine) orally or by intramuscular route. Dosage varies from 50 to 400 mg daily followed by maintenance doses of 25 mg twice a day. During early administration of chlorpromazine, hospitalization is recommended because of secondary blood pressure changes that can occur; however, complications from chlorpromazine are controllable and not serious.

Insofar as sympathetic discharges are thought to originate in the midbrain, a "short-circuiting" into the sensory nerve of the peripheral nerves is thought to be a sequence of the etiologic injury. Chlorpromazine is considered to act at the central level.

To minimize venous congestion and stasis edema, isometric muscular contraction should be started immediately. This type of exercise does not move the involved joints or elongate the inflamed tissues, but does cause the muscles to enhance venous return and mobilize the lymphatic circulation, thus removing the edema. Uninvolved joints must be actively moved through the full range of motion frequently during waking hours.

When unbearable pain prevents the patient's cooperation, the cervicothoracic sympathetic innervation must be interrupted. This can be done by blocking the stellate ganglion with procaine hydrochloride (Novocain) or one of its derivatives. On rare occasions in which a chemical block is effective but its benefit is of short duration, a surgical interruption of the sympathetic nerves is indicated. This intervention is rarely required. Even successful interruption of the sympathetic innervation does not permit the neglect of active motion, elevation, pain medication, and tranquilizers. *Cure cannot be achieved without patient cooperation.*

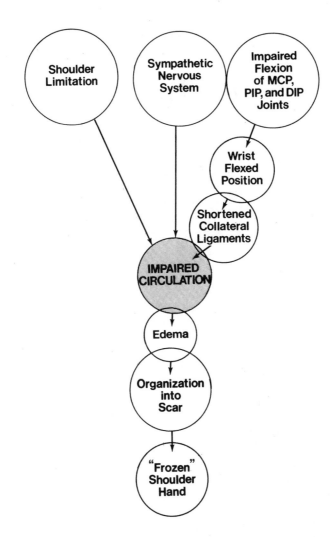

FIGURE 92. Sequences leading to "frozen" shoulder-hand-finger syndrome.

The presence of secondary gains when the alleged injury is industrial or a compensable personal injury adds a different factor. Pathologic malingering has not been clarified medically as either conscious or unconscious, but the end result is that the patient has a residual disability and has expended large financial sums. Treatment is identical medically but, to be effective, the motivation of secondary gains by maintaining the disability must be removed.

105

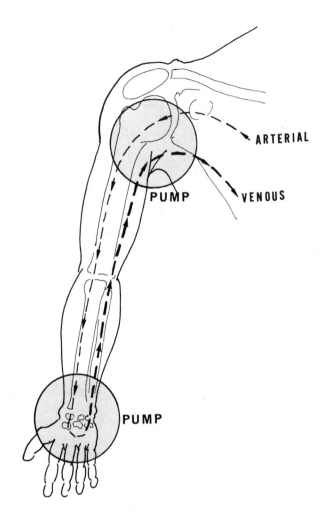

FIGURE 93. Venous lymphatic pumps of the upper extremity.

SHOULDER-HAND-FINGER SYNDROME

The shoulder-hand-finger syndrome is characteristic of the *minor* reflex sympathetic dystrophies. The causes are more discernible than those of causalgia. Some causes are as follows:

1. Postfracture (for example, Colles').
2. Posthemiparesis from cerebrovascular accident.
3. Postmyocardial infarction.
4. Postcast compression.

106

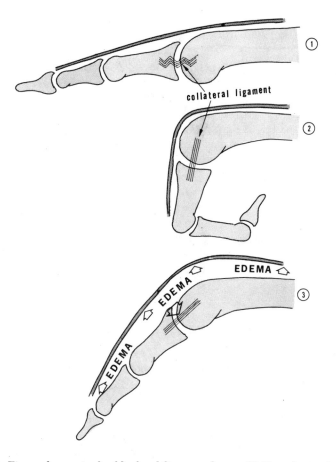

FIGURE 94. Finger changes in shoulder-hand-finger syndrome. *(1)* Normal extension of the metacarpophalangeal joint. Collateral ligaments are relaxed. *(2)* In normal flexion, the collateral ligaments become taut. *(3)* Edema occurs on the dorsum of the finger elevating the extensor tendons; this prevents flexion. The collateral ligaments become elevated in the extended finger position, causing them to be taut and preventing flexion.

5. Postinjection.
6. Postshoulder peritendonitis, bursitis, or fracture.

In fact, almost any trauma, major or minor, has been incriminated as inciting an etiology sequence dependent upon the initial site of the syndrome: shoulder, wrist, or fingers (Fig. 92). Once initiated, it may progress proximally or distally to ultimately become a "full blown" entity.

In the hand, the initial observable tissue reaction is dorsal edema of the fingers. The skin becomes smooth and shiny. The dorsal wrinkles over the knuckles and the fingers become obliterated (as compared with the oppo-

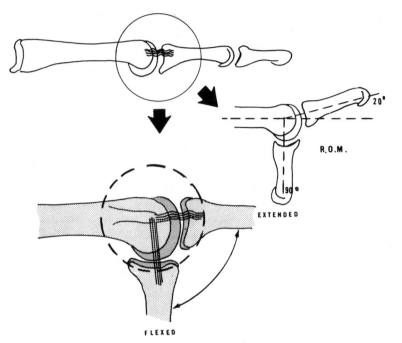

FIGURE 95. Normal flexion-extension of the metacarpophalangeal joints. Owing to the elliptical shape of the head of the metacarpals, the collateral ligaments are slack when the fingers are extended and taut when the fingers are flexed.

site normal hand). There is some edema, which may be pitting. As a result of the edema under (thus elevating) the extensor tendons, flexion of the fingers is limited. The "pump" action of the hand is impaired and more edema results (Fig. 93).

Edema seeps under the collateral ligaments, making them taut (Fig. 94). Because the collateral ligaments of the extended fingers must be relaxed to permit digital flexion (Fig. 95), their becoming taut further restricts flexion and further impairs pumping action. If there is simultaneous limited movement of the shoulder, the shoulder pump (glenohumeral joint) does not remove the venous lymphatic fluid of the upper extremity and the antigravity position of the arm cannot be attained; thus, more edema of the hand ensues. Once established and uncorrected, the edema organizes; further contracture results once all the signs and symptoms, other than the causalgic (burning) symptoms ensue.

Treatment

Treatment of the shoulder-hand-finger syndrome depends upon early recognition at a time during which all tissue changes are still reversible

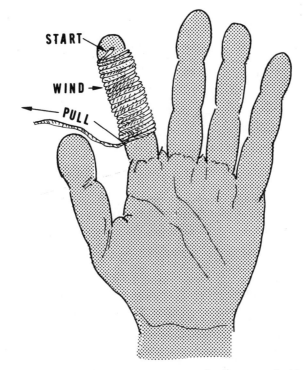

FIGURE 96. Removal of finger edema. Each finger is firmly wrapped with a heavy twine, beginning at the tip and moving toward the webbing. This procedure should be performed several times daily and can frequently be done by the patient using the uninvolved upper extremity.

and no permanent pathology has resulted. Essentially, treatment requires resumption of the shoulder-hand-finger pumps with restoration of anti-gravity forces. The techniques and objectives of treatment are as follows:

1. Return of glenohumeral range of motion.
2. Elevation of the arm-hand above the cardiac level to ensure gravity drainage.
3. Active wrist-finger-hand flexion exercises.
4. Passive mobilization of all joints involved; that is, the glenohumeral joint of the shoulder complex, the wrist (carporadial), the metacarpophalangeal joint, and the interphalangeal joint.
5. Mechanical removal of fluid from fingers and hand by compression "wrap dressing" (Fig. 96).[3]
6. Jobst-type of vasopneumatic compression to arm.
7. Stellate anesthetic blocks, of value in the presence of pain attributable to the sympathetic nervous system (causalgia).

REFERENCES

1. Homans, J.: Minor causalgia: A hyperesthetic neurovascular syndrome. N. Engl. J. Med. 222:870, 1940.
2. Mitchell, S. W., Moorehouse, G. R., and Kean, W. W.: Gunshot Wounds and Other Injuries of Nerves. J. B. Lippincott, Philadelphia, 1964.
3. Cain, H. D. and Liebgold, H. B.: Compressive centripetal wrapping technic for reduction of edema. Archives of Physical Medicine 48:420, 1967.

BIBLIOGRAPHY

Dabbs, C. H., and Peirce, E. C.: Causalgia treated with chlorpromazine hydrochloride. J.A.M.A. 159:1626, 1955.

Doupe, J., Culler, C. H., and Chance, G. Q.: Post-traumatic pain and the causalgic syndrome. J. Neurol. Neurosurg. Psychiatry 7:33, 1944.

Dundee, J. W.: Chlorpromazine as an adjunct in the relief of chronic pain. Br. J. Anaesth. 29:28, 1957.

Gilliat, R. W. and Wilson, T. G.: A pneumatic tourniquet test in the carpal tunnel syndrome. Lancet 2:595, 1953.

Hale, M. S.: A Practical Approach to Arm Pain. Charles C Thomas, Springfield, Ill., 1971.

Magee, R. B. and Palen, G. W.: Tardy ulnar palsy. Am. J. Surg. 78:470, 1949.

Mayfield, F. H.: Causalgia. Charles C Thomas, Springfield, Ill., 1951.

Shaw, R. S.: Pathological malingering. N. Engl. J. Med. 271:22, 1964.

Steinbrocker, O. and Lapin, L.: Reflex Dystrophy: Reflex Dystrophy in the Extremities. Rheumatic Diseases: Proc. of the 7th Int. Cong. on Rheumatic Diseases. W. B. Saunders, Philadelphia, 1952.

Sudeck, P.: Veber die acute Enzundicke Knochenatrophie. Arch. f. Klin. Chir. 62:147, 1900.

Volkmann, A. W.: Die ischaemischen Mushellahnungen. Zentralbe. Chir. 51:801, 1881.

CHAPTER 4

Tendons: Injuries and Diseases

Pain and impairment of the hand can result from injury to, infection of, and severance of the tendons. As with other tissues of the hand, knowledge of functional anatomy is essential for proper diagnosis and treatment.

TENDON SEVERANCE

Severance of tendons results in loss of motion of the joints involved. Treatment is surgical after certain basic guidelines have been observed. The decision of initial (primary) suture, rather than secondary suture after intentional delay, depends upon the site of the laceration and the function of the tendon.

Extensor Tendons

The extensor tendons do not usually retract after being severed; thus they can be sutured soon after the injury. The severed extensor tendon must be kept sutured for three to four weeks; therefore, the suture material should not be absorbable and should ultimately be easily withdrawn. Stainless steel is preferable to silk, which cannot be pulled through tissues after three weeks.

The ends of severed tendons, once they are approximated, go through various stages of healing. During the first two to three days, there is an outpouring of fibrin. By the fifth day, this fibrin mass is invaded by fibroblasts, which form fibrils that fuse into long threads. These threads merge into bundles that bridge the gap between the tendon ends. By the third week, edema and increased vascularity are decreased and there is a sufficiently strong union to permit traction upon the tendon. These factors are the reasons for three weeks of immobilization following tendon repair.

111

Tendons contained *within* a sheath, when severed, show more deterioration and heal more slowly than those without sheaths. The swelling that occurs within the sheath apparently obstructs venous return and impairs tendon nutrition and healing.

Adhesions that form around a healing tendon present a serious impairment to function after healing is complete. Numerous approaches, such as wrapping the tendon in cellophane, local or parenteral steroids, and insertion of tubules of various materials around the tendons, have been tried to prevent these adhesions. None has been effective to date.

The technique of suturing tendons is beyond the scope of this book but is well documented in the literature. The ends of the severed tendon must be approximated, and after suture the wrist must be immobilized for three to five weeks with 30 to 40° extension with the fingers also extended. This position of immobilization for sutured extensor tendons violates the general principle of immobilizing the hand in the *position of function*, with the wrist slightly extended and the fingers flexed. Sutured extensor tendons, however, usually result in good function.

The extensor pollicis longus retracts a considerable distance. The site of division of this tendon should not be laid wide open in an attempt to find the proximal segment. Rather, a proximal incision above the wrist should be made. When the tendon is located there, it can be passed through its passage by use of a smooth probe.

Flexor Tendons

Suturing of a severed flexor tendon in so-called "no man's land" (Fig. 97) has an unfavorable prognosis. This is due to the anatomic arrangement of the tendons in this area. A sutured tendon usually swells and this area has no room for expansion. Ischemic necrosis results.

When a tendon is divided in no man's land, primary suture should be avoided. Primary care should concern the wound with tendon transplant undertaken four to five weeks after the injury. Primary suture of the severed tendon in this zone not only gives poor results but often interferes with the ultimate graft procedure.

Flexor tendons severed *distal* to no man's land (the profundus tendons) can be primarily sutured. In this situation, the distal portion of the tendon usually is surgically removed from the site of insertion and the proximal tendon stump is attached to the site of the old insertion. Shortening as much as one-half inch of the reattached profundus does not interfere with the uninjured superficialis function.

Flexor tendons that are cut *proximal* to no man's land, especially injuries at the level of the wrist, can be sutured with good functional results. Attempts to resuture tendons individually, for example, profundus to profundus or superficialis to superficialis, usually result in functional failure.

112

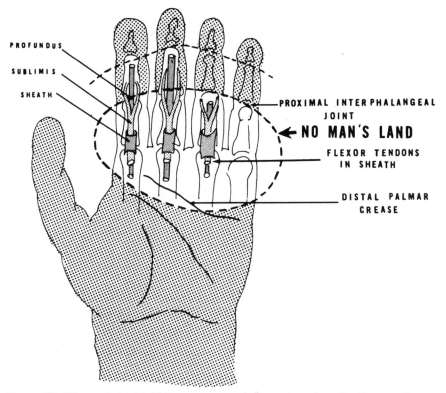

PROFUNDUS

SUBLIMIS

SHEATH

PROXIMAL INTERPHALANGEAL
JOINT

← NO MAN'S LAND

FLEXOR TENDONS
IN SHEATH

DISTAL PALMAR
CREASE

FIGURE 97. "No man's land." This area represents the region where the flexor tendons (profundus and sublimis) are tightly enclosed within a sheath. Primary repair of tendons in this region is *contraindicated*. Suture of the skin should be contemplated. Primary suture between the two interphalangeal joints should be avoided because the tendon inserts in this region.

Usually, only the profundus tendon is repaired. Because the profundus flexes the distal interphalangeal joint, good finger flexion results. When the superficialis tendon is severed, it is usually excised several millimeters from its attachment into the middle phalanx and allowed to retract. Suture of the cut flexor tendon of the thumb (flexor pollicis) usually gives good functional results.

After flexor tendon repair, the hand is immobilized for three weeks in slight wrist flexion with flexion of the involved finger or fingers. *The uninvolved fingers should not be immobilized.*

TENDON RUPTURE

A tendon may be ruptured from an acute stretch injury. The tendon normally is the strongest portion of the musculotendinous-osseous link

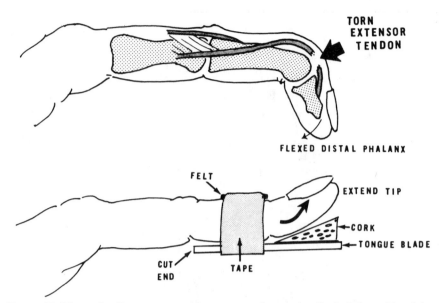

FIGURE 98. The mallet finger, rupture of extensor tendon to the distal phalanx. Forceful flexion of the distal phalanx may tear the extensor tendon from the distal phalanx. The end of the finger remains in a flexed position and cannot be actively extended. Treatment consists of immobilizing the finger with the distal phalanx in *hyper*extension for five to six weeks. The splint shown is a tongue blade reaching only to the middle phalangeal joint. A wedge of cork is glued to the blade and the finger is taped to the splint with a piece of felt inserted to protect the dorsum of the finger.

and therefore seldom tears. Tearing at its insertion occurs, with or without avulsion of the bone. Lesser stress may rupture a diseased or frayed tendon. Rheumatoid synovitis and fraying or moving over a rough bone fragment make a tendon particularly susceptible to rupture.

Mallet finger is caused by a forceful flexion injury to the distal phalanx during an activity in which the extensor tendon is taut, as in catching a baseball. The extensor tendon is torn from its insertion into the distal phalanx and in 25 percent of cases, a piece of bone is avulsed with it (Fig. 98). Clinically, the tip of the finger drops and extension is not possible.

Usually, conservative treatment results in good function within five weeks by immobilizing the distal phalanx in hyperextension. There are numerous ideas regarding the best manner of immobilization, ranging from casting the entire hand with the distal joint in hyperextension and the proximal joints flexed to merely splinting the distal joint (see Fig. 98). By flexing the middle phalanx, the central extensor slip will pull the extensor mechanism distally and allow the tear to unite. The lateral bands are also relaxed by this position (Fig. 99). If treatment is begun within ten days of injury, it can be cast as shown in Figure 100 for five

114

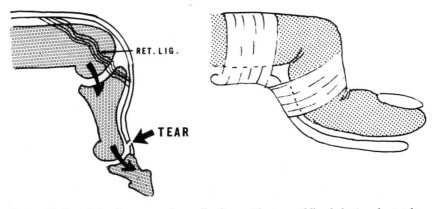

FIGURE 99. Rationale of treatment for mallet finger. Flexing middle phalanx and extending the distal digit permits the extensor tendon to unite. This position pulls the extensor mechanism distally and relaxes the lateral bands.

weeks followed by splinting of the distal joint for another four weeks. A short splint is worn for two more months to improve extension if there is pain, soreness, or functional impairment. If the proximal joints are stiff from previous treatment, this takes precedence in treatment and the flexed distal digit is ignored. Surgery is indicated when the residual functional impairment is unacceptable.

A fracture of the proximal portion of the distal phalanx, which clinically resembles mallet finger, must not be immobilized in extension, since the resultant extended distal phalanx will have a greater disabling deformity. Open reduction of such a fracture is indicated.

Extensor Tendon Rupture at Middle Phalanx

Rupture of the insertion of the extensor tendon into the middle pha-

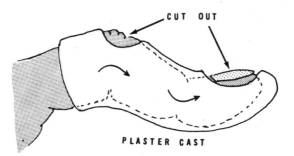

FIGURE 100. Plaster cast treatment for mallet finger. The cast holds the distal joint hyperextended and the middle joint flexed. The dorsum of the middle joint and the nail are exposed.

115

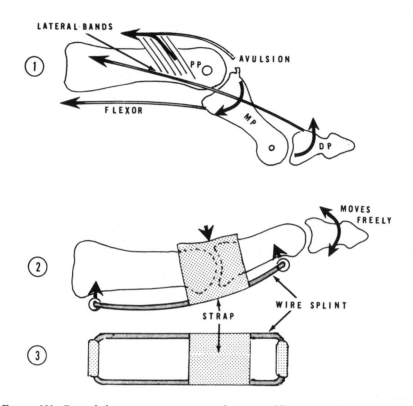

FIGURE 101. Buttonhole rupture, extensor tendon at middle joint, split treatment. *(1)* Avulsion of the extensor tendon permits the lateral bands to move in a palmar direction, pulling in a proximal direction. The flexor tendons now flex the middle phalanx (MP) and the lateral bands extend the distal phalanx (DP). *(2)* The splint is made of firm wire bent to extend the middle joint. The strap is inelastic. The distal phalanx is left free and motion is encouraged. *(3)* Dorsal view of the splint.

lanx, with or without bony avulsion, can occur from a direct blow or crushing injury. The injury may also attenuate the tendon, permitting a subsequent forceful flexion to cause it to rupture.

Rupture of the middle slip of the extensor mechanism allows the lateral slips to move in a palmar direction (Fig. 101) below the axis of joint rotation of the proximal and middle phalanges (PP and MP in Fig. 101). Combining with the action of the flexor superficialis, the proximal interphalangeal joint flexes and the lateral slips extend the distal phalanx. Any flexion activity further separates the torn tendon, thus preventing its union. Active extension of the finger also separates the severed tendon by applying tension upon the lateral slip.

Initially, in this tendon rupture, swelling and pain occur and all motion is restricted. Several days after the injury, the diagnosis becomes more

116

evident. Flexion of the finger at all joints now becomes possible, but extension of the middle phalanx (middle joint) is restricted. If the middle joint is passively held in full extension, the spasm and retraction of the interossei prevent full flexion of the distal joint.

Treatment consists of splinting the middle joint in hyperextension and leaving the distal joint free (see Fig. 101). This splint can be made of firm wire fashioned in the shape of a paper clip, with the finger held by a nonelastic strap. The splint is worn constantly for five weeks during which time the patient is instructed to *actively* flex the distal joint forcefully and frequently. When the distal joint can be flexed fully, it may be assumed that the intrinsic muscles are back in balance and that the extensor apparatus is reattached. The splint can then be removed. Surgical repair may be indicated (Fig. 102) when there is a bony avulsion or when the tendon tear has been of long duration before treatment is instituted. Normally, early diagnosis and proper splinting result in good functional recovery.

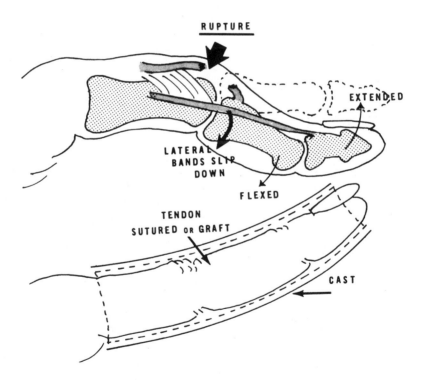

FIGURE 102. Extensor communis tear, surgical repair followed by plaster splint. The mechanism described in Figure 101 is shown. After surgical repair, the finger can be splinted as shown.

117

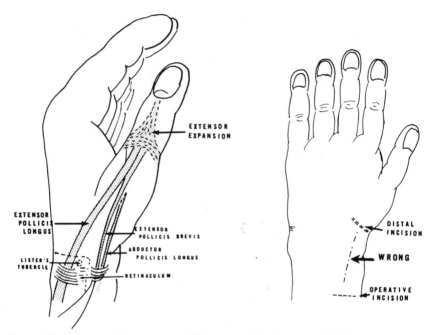

FIGURE 103. Rupture of the extensor pollicis longus. The extensor pollicis longus extends to the distal phalanx along a diagonal course. Its rupture results in loss of extension of the distal digit of the thumb, and some weakness of extension of the proximal joint. The ruptured tendon retracts considerably. End-to-end suture is not feasible, and grafting is required. Rather than extending the laceration, a proximal incision to locate the distal tendon must be made, and the graft is then passed through the canal with a smooth probe.

Extensor Pollicis Longus Rupture

The extensor pollicis longus tendon curves around the dorsal radial tubercle of Lister (Fig. 103), passes over the radial wrist extensors, and continues on to the thumb. At the point where the tendon angulates, wear and tear of the tendon occur. A Colles' fracture in particular can weaken this ligament. Rupture of this ligament results in the inability to extend the distal joint of the thumb and in weakness of extension of the proximal joint. Normally, the tendon can be palpated when the wrist is extended and the thumb is abducted.

Primary suture of the two fragmented ends is *not possible*, since it will neither hold nor function. Treatment requires surgical grafting of the severed tendon from a site proximal to the dorsal retinaculum to the end located at the metacarpal. It may be necessary to transfer the tendon of the extensor indicis. If grafting is done, a splint must be worn for one month.

118

Rupture of Flexor Tendons

Flexor tendons usually rupture when the tendons are diseased. Hyperextension of the fingers or forceful flexion against resistance is the usual history (50 percent of cases). Many patients with this condition, however, do not give a history of injury.

Treatment of one or more torn flexor tendons depends upon the site of the rupture and the degree of disability, as well as the underlying disease of the tendon. It is often best *not* to treat this type of rupture because the treatment may cause more residual disability than does the rupture.

TENDON DISEASES

Tenosynovitis

Excessive repetitive movement or unphysiologic stress of the tendon may inflame the tendon sheaths and cause painful impairment of motion. The symptoms include pain during any motion involving the tendon. The tendons are swollen and crepitation can be elicited during motion. The tendons most commonly involved are the dorsal extensors of the wrist, the extensor carpi ulnaris, and the long abductor and short extensor of the thumb (de Quervain's disease). Treatment consists of resting the part by splint or casting. Occasionally steroid injection is beneficial.

de Quervain's Disease

Stenosing tenosynovitis of the thumb abductors at the radiostyloid process is so prevalent that it merits special mention. This disease was named after the Swiss surgeon de Quervain,[1] who described the condition in 1895.

The tendons of the abductor pollicis longus and the extensor pollicis brevis usually move in the same synovial sheath (Fig. 104) that passes in a bony groove over the radiostyloid process and, from there, forms a sharp angle of as much as 105°. Synovitis results from friction between the tendon, the sheath, and the bony process. This friction occurs during pinching with the thumb and simultaneous motion of the wrist. During pinching, the abductor pollicis longus stabilizes the thumb.

Symptoms of aching discomfort are localized over the styloid process with radiation into the hand or up the forearm. Aching or pain is aggravated by movements of the wrist and thumb. Characteristic symptoms can be reproduced by flexing the thumb and cupping it under the fingers, then flexing the wrist in an ulnar direction which stretches the thumb tendons. Abduction of the thumb against resistance also can reproduce

119

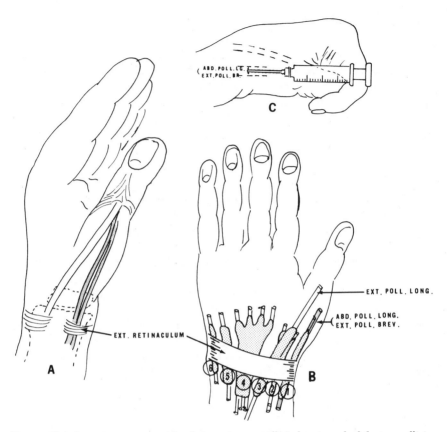

FIGURE 104. Stenosing tenosynovitis of the extensor pollicis brevis and abductor pollicis longus, de Quervain's disease. (A) The tendons pass over the prominence of the radial styloid process. The extensor pollicis longus tendon forms the ulnar border of the snuff box. (B) The six tendon sheaths pass under the extensor retinaculum. (1) and (3) are labeled, (2) contains the tendon of the extensor carpi radialis, (4) the extensor digitorum communis, (5) the extensor digiti minimi, and (6) the extensor carpi ulnaris. Tenosynovitis occurs commonly only at (1). (C) Method and site of injection of steroids in this condition.

the symptoms. There may be tenderness over the tendon but crepitation is rare.

The pathology takes the form of an increased vascularity of the outer sheath that, coupled with edema, thickens the sheath and constricts the enclosed tendon. The synovial fluid of the sheath increases and turns a yellowish color. Fine hair-like adhesions may be found between the sheath and the tendon and the sheath may be thickened to two to four times its normal size.

Treatment requires immobilization in a padded half-cast with injections of cortisone into the sheath. If there is no relief after four weeks of treatment, surgical decompression must be considered. Incision must not be longitudinal along the tendon sheath because an incision in this direction can cause a scar or keloid. A transverse incision, followed by undermining the skin, then a longitudinal incision of the overlying fascia and the sheath will adequately decompress the tendon. Both tendons (abductor pollicis longus and extensor pollicis brevis) must be within the sheath or the decompression procedure will not relieve the symptoms.

Trigger Thumb

In this condition, the thumb snaps as it flexes and may become locked in flexion or in extension. This situation occurs from thickening of the sheath or the tendon, or both, which prevents gliding of the tendon within the sheath. A nodule can form on the tendon which prevents the tendon from passing through the sheath at the metacarpal head.

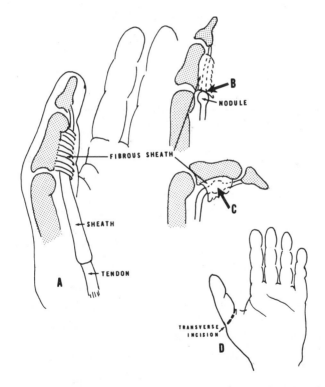

FIGURE 105. Trigger thumb, snapping thumb flexor. (A) The relationship of the flexor tendon within its bursa sheath covered by a fibrous sheath canal. (B) A nodular thickening of the tendon prevents flexion. (C) The nodule is trapped under the sheath and re-extension is prevented. (D) The site and direction of skin incision decompresses the tenosynovitis.

121

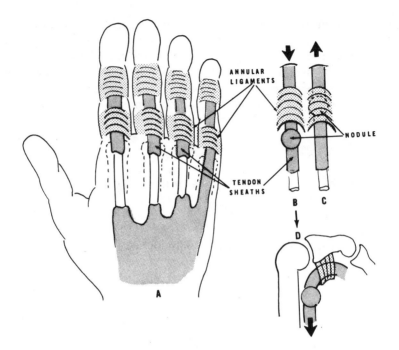

FIGURE 106. Trigger fingers. The anatomy of the flexor region. *(A)* The flexor tendon within its synovial sheath passes under the annular ligament at the metacarpal head. *(B)* The fusiform swelling of the tendon plus thickening of the sheath proximal to the ligament. When it swells and gets in the position *(D)*, re-extension *(C)* is prevented.

Local injections of cortisone into the sheath may result in good recovery; if locking persists, excision of the thickened sheath is easily performed. The sheath is reached through a *transverse* incision at the crease over the metacarpal head (Fig. 105).

Trigger Fingers

Snapping flexor tendons or trigger fingers consist of a sudden snapping sensation of the finger during flexion and re-extension. Flexion is restricted; then the finger suddenly flexes to be locked in flexion and is unable to be actively re-extended. This occurs most frequently in the middle or ring fingers and is attributed to direct, severe, or multiple trauma to the flexor portion of the fingers. Injury pinches the flexor tendon and its sheath between the head of the metacarpal and the bruising object. The trauma may be acute and severe, or repetitive.

The ligamentous sheath (Fig. 106) thickens. The tendon enlarges into a fusiform swelling and forms a nodule within its thickened synovium-lined sheath. The nodule moves within the ligamentous sheath until the nodule is too thick or the sheath too constricted, then obstruction occurs. The site of the nodule determines whether or not the finger can actively flex or is locked and cannot re-extend.

Cortisone injections into the sheath may relieve the obstruction. If this fails, a transverse incision proximal to the palpable nodule exposes the annular band, which then is merely slit. Excision of the nodule invariably causes a new and bigger nodule to form.

Dupuytren's Contracture

Dupuytren's contracture is a fibrous contracture of the palmar fascia

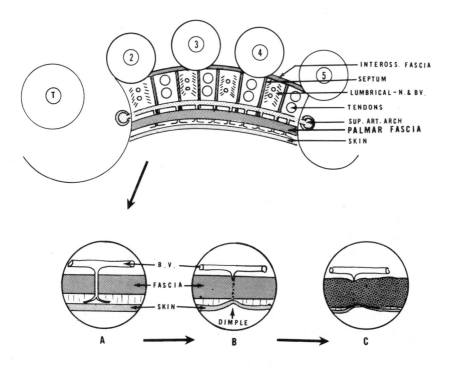

FIGURE 107. Dupuytren's contracture. The upper picture shows the normal anatomy of the palmar fascia. The palmar skin is firmly attached with little subcutaneous fat. Fibrous septa penetrate to the deep interosseous fascia and form spaces. These eight compartments contain the flexor tendons with the alternate compartments containing the lumbrical muscles and neurovascular elements. The skin receives its blood supply by vessels from the superficial arch which penetrates through the fascia. (A) An enlargement of the normal palm. (B) Thickening of the fascia constricting the penetrating nutrient artery. The skin puckers to form the characteristic dimple. (C) The fascia ultimately becomes markedly thickened and contracted and the overlying skin atrophic.

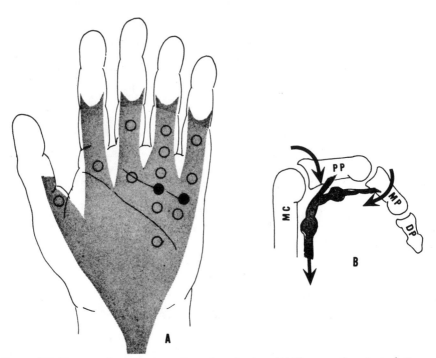

FIGURE 108. Dupuytren's contracture, site and mechanism. *(A)* These are the principal sites where nodules form in the palmar fascia. The fourth and fifth fingers are most frequently involved. *(B)* The fascial slips extend to the second phalanx (MP). When they shorten because of contracture, they cause flexion deformity of the metacarpophalangeal or proximal interphalangeal joints, or both.

with ultimate flexion contractures of the fingers at the metacarpophalangeal and proximal interphalangeal joints. The condition was first described by Clive in 1808, but Dupuytren[2] first described an operation for its treatment and his name has become associated with it.

For no known reason, the palmar fascia thickens and contracts. It is a disease found in Caucasian men in their fifth to seventh decades. There is no association with occupation, but there is a strong association with epilepsy and an increase with chronic invalidism such as pulmonary tuberculosis and alcoholism.

The palmar fascia covers the palm of the hand. It extends proximally as a continuation of the palmaris longus tendon, passing distally into the fingers and ultimately attaching to the sides of the proximal and middle phalanges (see Figs. 32 and 33). In the palmar region, the skin is firmly attached to the fascia by numerous fasciculi with scant subcutaneous fat.

The undersurface of the palmar fascia passes into the depth of the palm by perpendicular fibrous septa. These septa form eight longitudinal compartments alternately containing the flexor tendons and the neurovascu-

124

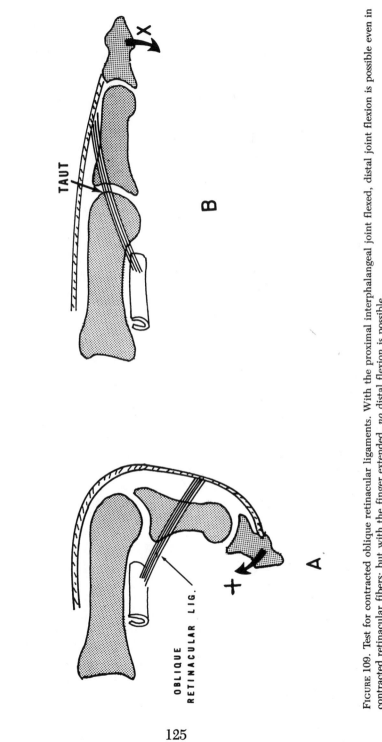

FIGURE 109. Test for contracted oblique retinacular ligaments. With the proximal interphalangeal joint flexed, distal joint flexion is possible even in contracted retinacular fibers; but with the finger extended, *no* distal flexion is possible.

lar bundles and lumbrical muscles (Fig. 107). The palmar skin receives its circulation from tiny branches of the superficial volar arch (see Fig. 89) which penetrates the palmar fascia. As the fascia undergoes fibrosis, thickens, and contracts, it pulls upon the tiny fasciculi connected to the skin causing the skin to *dimple*. Further thickening of the fascia occludes the circulation and the skin atrophies. This explains the poor postoperative healing. The palmar fascia thickening involves the perpendicular septa and distally the longitudinal bands that pass over the metacarpal heads and attach to the base of the phalanges. As the fascia fibrosis contracts, it forms nodules and the fingers develop flexion contracture (Fig. 108). Stretching of the fascia by extension of the finger joints causes the involved longitudinally oriented fibers to react by contraction and further hypertrophy.

Symptoms usually consist of *painless* thickening of the palmar skin and underlying fascia with either dimpling or formation of nodules. The initial site is usually near the distal palmar crease (see Fig. 91). Although any of the digits can be involved, the ring and little fingers are most commonly affected. Forty percent of patients have the condition bilaterally. Handedness is not relevant.

Flexion contracture gradually develops in the fingers at the metacarpophalangeal and proximal interphalangeal joints. Symptoms take the form of functional disability and disturbing appearance, but pain is rare. The fibrous band along the palmar aspect of the fingers with limited digit extension is characteristic.

Since hypertrophy is caused by stress, release of the stress decreases the fibrous hypertrophy. Release may be accomplished by merely excising the fascial bands—simple incision release of skin and fascia followed by skin graft insertion. The fascia that is incised is limited or confined to the palmar fascia and the contracted digit. The depth of the excision is limited to the more superficial longitudinal fascial bundles and transverse interdigital fibers. The transverse palmar hands are not involved and thus are not interrupted.

Preservation of skin blood supply, atraumatic dissection, closure without tension, absolute hemostasis, and early immobilization are the criteria of successful surgery. Contracture of the oblique retinacular ligament may occur from Dupuytren's contracture. This can be tested, as illustrated in Figure 109.

Nonoperative treatment is being revived for Dupuytren's contracture. Injection of trypsin, chymotrypsin A, hyaluronidase, and lidocaine followed by forceful extension of the finger ruptures the skin and contracted fascia. Both of these ultimately heal with good finger range of motion. This nonoperative treatment is recommended in elderly patients or in those unfit for surgery.

126

REFERENCES

1. de Quervain, F.: Korresp. Bl. Schweiz. Arz. 25:389, 1895.
2. Dupuytren, G.: Clinical lectures on surgery, delivered at Hotel Dieu in 1832. Translated by A. S. Doane. Collins and Hannay, New York 1833.

BIBLIOGRAPHY

Bassot, J.: Traitment de las maladie de Dupuytren par exercise pharmaco-dynamic base physiologique technique. Gaz. Hop. 16:557, 1969.

Boyes, J. H.: Bunnell's Surgery of the Hand, ed. 3. J. B. Lippincott, Philadelphia, 1956.

Boyle, J. R.: Dupuytren's contracture. Etiology and principles of treatment. California Medicine 110:292, 1969.

Chase, R. A.: Surgery of the hand. 1. N. Engl. J. Med. 287:1174, 1972.

Finklestein, H.: Stenosing tendovaginitis at the radial styloid process. J. Bone Joint Surg. 12:509, 1930.

Gonzalez, R. I.: A simplified surgical approach in the treatment of Dupuytren's contracture. In: Cramer, L. M. and Chase, R. A. (eds.): Symposium of the Hand, Vol. 3. C. V. Mosby, St. Louis, 1971, p. 123.

Hueston, J. T.: Dupuytren's Contraction. Williams & Wilkins, Baltimore, 1963.

Luck, J. V.: Dupuytren's contracture. J. Bone Joint Surg. 41-A:635, 1959.

Palmborg, G.: Stenosing tenosynovitis. Ann. Rheum. Dis. 11:193, 1952.

Rhode, C. M. and Jennings, W. D.: Dupuytren's contracture. Am. Surg. 33:855, 1967.

Skoog, T.: Dupuytren's contracture: With special reference to etiology and improved surgical treatment. Acta Chir. Scand. (Suppl.) 139:1, 1948.

CHAPTER 5

Fractures and Dislocations of the Finger and Hand

PRINCIPLES OF TREATMENT

Fractures and dislocations of the fingers have frequently been ignored even though trivial injuries have resulted in severe disability. The loss of finger function interferes markedly with the use of the entire upper extremity.

The following principles regarding the care of injured phalanges and interphalangeal joints must not be violated:

1. Immobilization must be instituted to relieve pain and permit primary healing. Active or passive motion will cause more, not less, stiffness. If tissues are torn, immobilization must be maintained at least for 10 to 14 days.
2. Immobilization must be maintained in flexion (Fig. 110). *No* fracture or dislocation of a finger requires maintenance of *extension of all three joints.* The splinting of the entire finger on a tongue blade or straight metal splint is to be discouraged.
3. All digits that need not be immobilized *must be actively mobilized.* Only the injured part of the finger should be splinted and all other joints of the finger moved actively and passively. If one finger is immobilized in complete extension, it is impossible to fully flex the other fingers. Joints must be *actively,* not passively, moved and stretched.
4. Swelling must be avoided by elevating the hand and *actively* moving the shoulder, elbow, wrist, and fingers frequently through their full range of motion.

Fractures of the phalanges must be reduced accurately. This requires recognizing the exact site of fracture and understanding the muscle pull

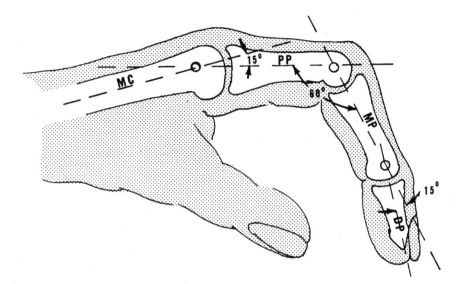

FIGURE 110. Position of immobilization of finger joints in treatment of fractures. Immobilization of the joints of the fingers in treatment of fractures is best done with 15° of the metacarpophalangeal joint, 60° at the proximal interphalangeal joint, and 15° at the distal joint.

upon the fragments, then minimizing this deforming force (Fig. 111).

Interphalangeal joint sprains thought to be *simple* or *mere strains* often are subluxations or self-reduced dislocations with capsular tears or minor avulsion fractures. Recognizing this possibility is important, since all sprains should be treated as dislocations or subluxations and should be splinted for two to three weeks in the flexed position, then actively exercised. Painless functional recovery is thus likely.

Fractures of the phalanges distal to the metacarpophalangeal joint have the tendency to displace because of musculotendinous pull on the fragments. With the probability of fragment displacement, immobilization by traction is advisable. Traction is not used for reduction of the fracture, but merely for immobilization of the phalanges in their proper position. Reduction is best done manually with the patient anesthetized or with an axillary block.

The duration of immobilization is *not equated with the time of healing,* but is *shorter* than that of healing. Active range-of-motion exercises must be started before x-ray films show evidence of healing. This is usually within one to two weeks. Prolonged immobilization is as detrimental as is excessive manipulation.

Moberg[1] has postulated comparative healing times (Fig. 112) claiming that the thinner distal portion of the phalanx is denser and less vascular and thus heals more slowly than the proximal portion and the proximal

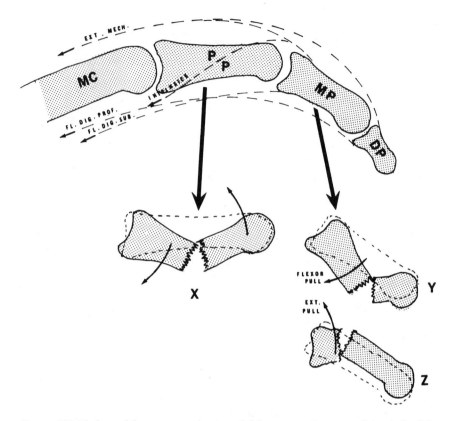

FIGURE 111. Phalangeal fractures, mechanism of deformation. Fractures of the shaft of the proximal phalanx (PP) bow in a palmar direction because of the pull of the intrinsics (lumbricals and interossei) which flex the proximal and extend the distal fragments (X). In fractures of the middle phalanx (MP) at the distal shaft (Y), the proximal fragment flexes because of the pull of the flexor tendons. In a fracture through the proximal shaft (Z), the extensor mechanism acting upon the distal fragment causes dorsal bowing. Regardless of the site or direction of bowing, the treatment consists of traction, reduction, and casting in the flexed position.

phalanx. The narrower distal portion on the middle phalanx heals in 10 to 14 weeks, the distal portion of the proximal phalanx in five to seven weeks, and the remainder of the finger in three to five weeks.

In open fractures, the wound should be excised immediately under strict sterile technique, and the wound should be covered as soon and as completely as possible. Early, if not immediate, amputation of a severely damaged or crushed digit is indicated if it can be reasonably estimated that the finger will be permanently stiff, insensitive, and useless. Infection of a mutilated finger with resultant stiffness of the other fingers is best treated by resection of the infected finger, thus preventing further

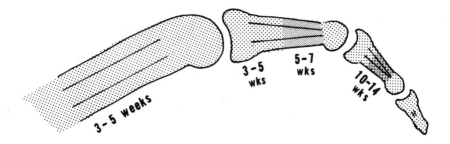

FIGURE 112. Fracture healing time. Bone relatively more vascular and cancellous heals more rapidly than denser bone. The former is found in the broader proximal portion of the phalanx and in the most proximal phalanx. The distal portion of the proximal phalanx consolidates in five to seven weeks, whereas the distal portion of the middle phalanx takes 10 to 14 weeks. It is not necessary to immobilize fractures for these lengths of time. (Modified after Moberg, E.: Emergency Surgery of the Hand. E & S Livingstone, London, 1967.)

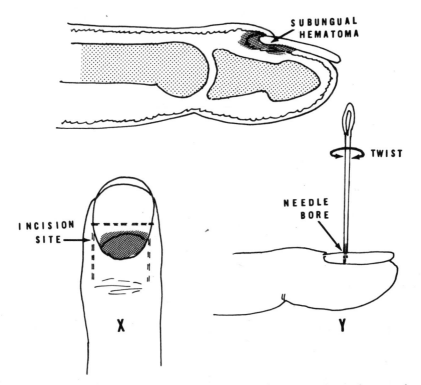

FIGURE 113. Evacuation of subungual hematoma. Upper figure shows the site of a post-traumatic hematoma. It can be evacuated by incising and elevating or removing the proximal half of the nail (X), or by boring a hole into the center of the hematoma with a needle heated to red-hot and twisted through the nail (Y).

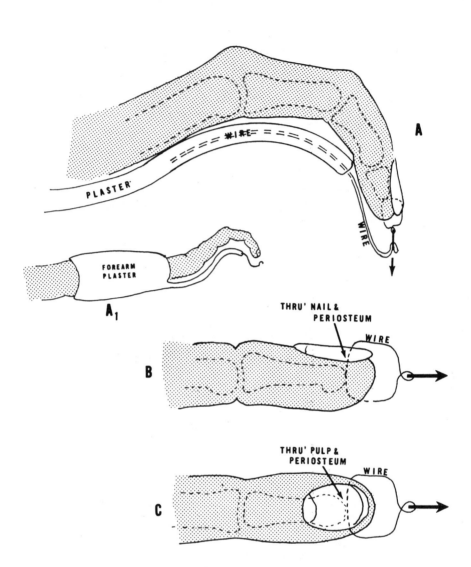

FIGURE 114. Fracture treatment with plaster traction. *(A)* A braided stainless steel suture (0.08 mm) or a traction pin can be inserted through the nail and distal phalanx periosteum *(B)* or through the pulp and periosteum *(C)* and traction applied by a wire incorporated into a flexed plaster cast. The cast extends to include the forearm *(A₁)*. Traction is used to immobilize, *not* to reduce, the fracture.

stiffness of the others. In children, amputation of a finger to avoid stiffness of the others should be delayed, since permanent residual stiffness is not predictable. The maxim of early amputation does not apply to the thumb, whose function must be salvaged as much as possible.

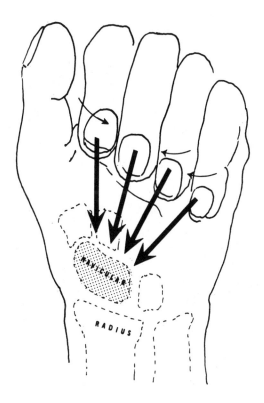

FIGURE 115. Direction of flexion immobilization in fractures of phalanges. The fingers normally flex across the palm in a direction towards the navicular (scaphoid) bone. The axis rotation about the middle finger (arrows) cannot be incorporated into casts or splints.

SPECIFIC SITES OF INJURY

Terminal Phalanx

Fractures of the terminal phalanx usually heal without incident unless there is avulsion of the extensor tendon (baseball finger) or a subungual hematoma (Fig. 113). Treatment of a fracture associated with a baseball finger that involves the distal joint should *not* include splinting in extension (the position for splinting the baseball finger), but rather splinting in the functional flexed position. A rigid distal phalanx in extension is more disabling than a flail flexed digit.

Subungual hematoma should be evacuated by lifting a flap of the nail or boring a hole directly through the nail with a red-hot needle (see Fig. 113).

133

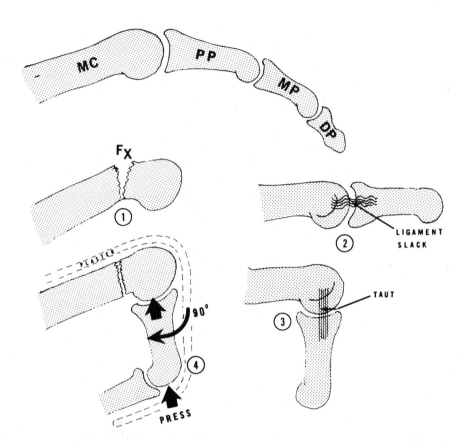

FIGURE 116. Fracture of neck of metacarpal. (1) The usual deformation of the distal fragment. (2) The lateral ligaments are slack when the proximal phalanx is extended so the fracture *cannot* be reduced in this position. (3) With the finger flexed, the metacarpophalangeal joint is immobile and the phalanx can be used to reduce the fracture which is then casted. (4) A dorsal splint applied for three weeks.

Middle Phalanx

Fracture of the middle phalanx tends to bow the finger because of the pull of the flexor digitorum sublimis on the proximal segment (see Fig. 111). Fracture of the proximal portion of the middle phalanx bows distally as a result of the pull of the extensor mechanism upon the distal fragment.

Treatment of phalanx fracture requires immobilization in flexion regardless of size and resultant deformity. If no displacement is evident, it is merely necessary to hold in a flexion splint, metal or plaster. If there is overriding or displacement, or both, manual reduction is indicated and the finger is then held by traction (Fig. 114). Use of adhesive traction requires careful frequent observation to avoid slipping or skin damage.

Immobilization of the fingers in flexion demands that the fingers be flexed toward the navicular (scaphoid) and not parallel to each other (Fig. 115). It is desirable that frequent x-rays be taken to ensure that there is no bowing so that the tendons are not compromised.

Immobilization should not exceed three weeks before active mobilization exercises are begun. A night splint for protection may be desired when a callus is not apparent at the fracture site. A fracture extending into a joint gives a poor prognosis, and immobilization in a flexed posture is necessary.

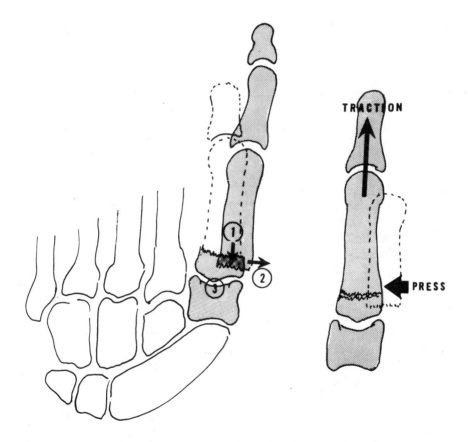

FIGURE 117. Simple impacted fracture of base of thumb metacarpal. Fracture of the base of the thumb metacarpal with impaction *(1)* and lateral displacement *(2)* but no involvement of the joint *(3)* is treated by reduction done with traction and simultaneous pressure against the distal fragment. The fracture is then casted.

Metacarpal

Fractures at the base of a metacarpal are usually innocuous and merely need dorsal splinting for three to four weeks with simultaneous active exercises of the fingers and thumb.

Fracture of the shaft requires reduction by manual manipulation with plaster immobilization that permits active motion of the fingers and the thumb. After manual reduction, if the fragments cannot be adequately held, then open reduction with the insertion of an intramedullary Kirschner wire may be desirable.

Fracture of the metacarpal neck requires manual manipulation for reduction, followed by casting for three weeks, then active exercises (Fig. 116). Fractures of metacarpals, especially with concomitant crush injuries, should *never* immobilize any of the digits or the metacarpophalangeal joint. This is especially true of black patients, who are more susceptible to scar or keloid formation. Active exercises must be instituted immediately and closely supervised. Physical therapy consisting merely of passive range of motion, whirlpool, and massage is ineffective. Patient participation in active exercises to use the full range of motion of each joint must be a full-time activity.

An Ace bandage must *not* be applied to the swollen hand. A bandage that can be placed so as to constrict at the wrist or the proximal hand will only increase distal swelling. Chronic edema will lead to fibrosis and a useless hand. During exercises and during much of the day, the hand is best elevated. A sling keeping the elbow flexed in an attempt to elevate the hand is to be avoided.

Dynamic splints under watchful care in a well-motivated patient may decrease the digit contractures, but they are not a substitute for frequent, *active* exercise.

Thumb

A frequent fracture site is the proximal metacarpal. These fractures (occurring mostly in men) result usually from direct blows to the thumb and are common in boxers. There are two major types of fractures of the base of the thumb: those that do not affect the joint, and those that are associated with dislocation of the carpometacarpal joint (Bennett fracture).

In a fracture of the base of the thumb without joint involvement, the fragments are angulated dorsally and are frequently impacted. Reduction is accomplished manually with simultaneous traction and pressure over the base (Fig. 117) and casting that includes the forearm and maintains the thumb slightly *ab*ducted with the metacarpophalangeal joint flexed. The distal joint of the thumb is kept free and active.

136

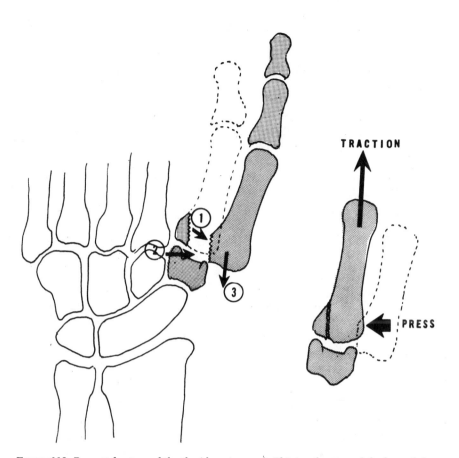

FIGURE 118. Bennett fracture of the thumb metacarpal. This is a fracture of the base of the thumb metacarpal with lateral displacement. *1* shows fracture through the base; *2* shows proximal disolcation; *3*, the dislocation is aggravated by the pull of the flexor and extensor tendons. This fracture is reduced by traction with simultaneous pressure against the distal fragment. Prognosis is guarded because of residual instability and ultimate degenerative arthritis.

A Bennett fracture occurs through the base of the thumb metacarpal separating a triangular fragment of the metacarpal. The metacarpal displaces laterally from the trapezium and moves upward (Fig. 118). The medial fragment is relatively unimportant. The metacarpal subluxes by sliding down the saddle-shaped trapezium, pulled proximally by the flexor and extensor tendons.

Base of the Fifth Metacarpal

Medial dislocation (in an ulnar direction) of the fifth metacarpal usually can be easily reduced; however, prevention of redislocation by hold-

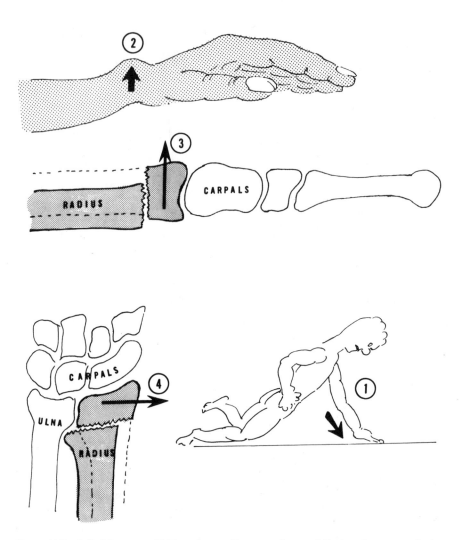

FIGURE 119. Colles' fracture. *(1)* Fracture usually occurs from a fall upon the outstretched hand. *(2)* The typical "dinner-fork" or "silver-fork" deformity is noted. *(3)* The distal fragment is displaced backward (dorsally) and *(4)* outward (radially).

ing may require skeletal fixation. Lateral dislocation (in a radial direction) across the palm requires open reduction.

Dislocations of the index, middle, and ring fingers are unusual, since these joints are relatively stable. Dislocation occurring either dorsally or towards the palm can be reduced by pressure upon the base with simultaneous traction. This is followed by a molded plaster cast for three weeks with simultaneous active exercises of the fingers.

138

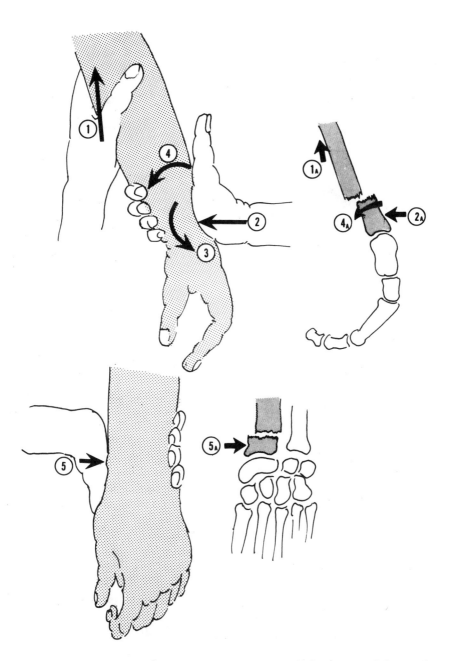

FIGURE 120. Reduction of Colles' fracture. (1) Traction is applied in a proximal direction by immobilizing the forearm with one hand. (2) The thenar eminence of the manipulating hand presses the radial fragment posteriorly causing (3) ulnar deviation. As the fragment slips into place, the forearm is (4) pronated. (5) A new grip is then taken and the fragment is pushed inward (ulnarly). The forearm is then casted in a carefully molded plaster.

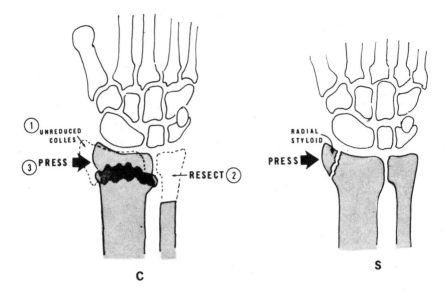

FIGURE 121. Treatment of an unreduced Colles' fracture; treatment of radial styloid fracture. *(C)* After six to eight weeks, the unreduced Colles' fracture cannot be reduced simply. The ulna can be resected, then the radial fragment can be manipulated into position. *(S)* If the styloid process of the radius can be reduced by direct pressure, it should be casted for four weeks.

Wrist

The most common fracture of the wrist is the *Colles'* fracture, in which a fracture through the radius causes the distal fragment to be displaced *radially and dorsally.* A "silver-fork" or "dinner-fork" deformity results (Fig. 119). This fracture usually occurs from a fall on the outstretched hand. Sprains of this joint are rare, but displacement of the radial epiphysis is common in children. What may be originally considered to be a sprain with a negative x-ray film should be viewed with suspicion, and x-ray examinations should be repeated in two to three weeks with oblique views to reveal concealed fractures.

Treatment demands complete correction, leaving no residual evidence of a fracture displacement. Failure to reduce the dorsal displacement or the radial displacement will leave disfigurement and often limitation of ulnar-radial movement.

Reduction by manipulation can be done in one manuever, but it is best done in two stages. The person performing the manipulation grasps the distal fragment (Fig. 120) with one hand (for example, the left hand for a right Colles' fracture), placing the thenar eminence of the manipulating hand over the radial fragment and the fingertips on the palmar side. The

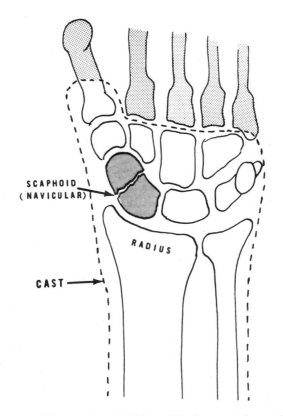

FIGURE 122. Fracture of the carpal scaphoid bone. This fracture is frequently missed on the initial x-ray examination and may require three views to reveal a hairline fracture. Suspicion is aroused by tenderness over the "snuff box," swelling, and painful wrist motion. The fracture should be treated by six to eight weeks of a snug plaster cast that includes the thumb metacarpal and extends to the carpometacarpal joints of the other fingers.

fragment is then pushed posteriorly. The opposite hand steadies the proximal forearm and permits traction. The manipulating hand can exert some pronation while forcing the distal fragment into place. After the dorsal dislocation is reduced, the hands are altered and the manipulating palm presses the fragment in an ulnar direction.

It is not possible to overcorrect a displacement by manual pressure. Only incomplete reduction can result. If the fracture is comminuted, complete reduction is mandatory and, in this situation, it may be necessary to compress the fragments between both thenar eminences of the manipulator.

After reduction, the wrist is immobilized in plaster that is applied while traction is maintained upon the patient's wrist by pulling on the thumb. The cast should extend from the upper forearm *to,* but *not in-*

141

cluding, the metacarpal heads. The wrist should be molded before the plaster sets.

The cast should be sufficiently snug to prevent displacement, but not so snug as to impair the circulation. In elderly people, the cast should be removed in 10 to 14 days and the wrist then placed in a more neutral position to prevent joint impairment.

It is imperative that active exercises be started immediately to assure complete range of motion of the fingers, thumb, elbow, and shoulder. These exercises must be started immediately after fracture reduction and must be done frequently, under daily supervision, if necessary, in the case of the reluctant patient. The arm should be elevated periodically to minimize edema. The cast should be maintained for four to five weeks. Earlier removal may permit displacement. A fracture that is unreduced after six to eight weeks cannot be reduced simply by manipulation, but can be reduced by excising the distal end of the ulna (Fig. 121). Fractures of the radial styloid process can be treated simply by manually compressing the fragment if there is displacement, then casting for four weeks (see Fig. 121).

A fall upon the outstretched arm causing forceful dorsiflexion of the wrist can cause a marginal fracture of the distal end of the radius that may be missed on original x-ray films. A repeat x-ray examination may reveal the fracture. This is an important fracture that may deform the groove in which the tendon of the flexor pollicis longus runs. If this fracture is not recognized, reduced, and immobilized, an irregularity that can fray the extensor tendon may result. Immobilization for two or three weeks with avoidance of thumb movement is necessary.

Injuries of the wrist demand x-ray films taken in three planes. The x-ray films should be examined with extreme care, and repeated films should be taken as desired to ascertain the presence of a fracture of the scaphoid (Fig. 122). Scaphoid bone fractures *never heal spontaneously* without prolonged, uninterrupted immobilization.

Symptoms of fractures of the scaphoid are pain, tenderness, and swelling in the "snuff box" after a fall on the outstretched hand. Movement of the wrist is painful. X-ray films must be taken in the anterior-posterior, lateral, and oblique views. Negative initial views *do not dispel* the diagnosis. If symptoms warrant, a diagnosis of fracture regardless of a negative x-ray treatment is justified. Only a negative x-ray result three to four weeks after the fall is conclusive.

Treatment requires *rigid* plaster immobilization extending from the metacarpals to the elbow and including the metacarpal of the thumb. The thumb metacarpal should be fully abducted with the interphalangeal joint slightly flexed. After three weeks, the cast can be removed and x-ray examination repeated. If then a fracture is revealed, the cast must be reapplied for a minimum of eight to ten weeks or when x-ray results show evidence of union. Union is verified if x-ray films reveal *obliteration* of the fracture line. Immobilization is the only effective treatment. Surgical intervention offers little help.

REFERENCE

1. Moberg, E.: Emergency Surgery of the Hand. E & S Livingstone, London, 1967.

CHAPTER 6

Joints: Injuries and Diseases

The study of joint injuries and diseases overlaps the topic of fractures and dislocations discussed in Chapter 5 by including dislocations as injuries to the soft tissues of the joints. Rheumatoid arthritis is primarily a disease of the soft tissue and ultimately manifests itself as joint deformity with pain and functional impairment. All are included in this chapter because of the similarities in structural changes and symptoms.

SPRAINS

Many sprains are momentary subluxations that spontaneously reduce. They escape detection on x-ray examination and tend to be ignored or minimized. They should be diagnosed as *reduced subluxations* and, barring complications, treated by immobilization in a slightly flexed position of function for a period of two to three weeks followed by progressive active exercises. Limitation and swelling may persist for months following sprain.

In a subluxation, as in a complete dislocation, the capsule and collateral ligaments may be torn, but to a lesser degree. A capsular tear in which the head of a metacarpal or phalanx herniates may cause reduction to be difficult and the prevention of recurrence after reduction equally difficult. Effective treatment of this type of problem requires open reduction and surgical repair of the tear in the capsule.

Interphalangeal and metacarpophalangeal dislocations are usually caused by hyperextension injuries. Reduction is possible by traction with simultaneous slight flexion followed by immobilization of that joint in slight flexion (Fig. 123). The metacarpophalangeal thumb joint is the digit most subject to dislocation. The proximal phalanx usually displaces backwards (dorsally) and the head of the metacarpal may protrude through the associated capsular tear. The capsule and the flexor tendons "buttonhole" the head of the metacarpal and maintain the dislocation

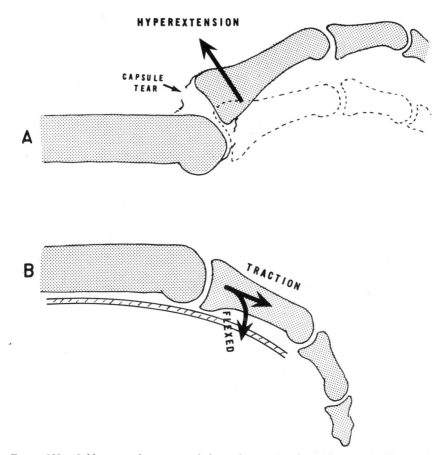

FIGURE 123.   Subluxation of metacarpophalangeal joint. *(A)* The mechanism of subluxation from a hyperextension injury in which the capsule may be torn and the head of the metacarpal or the base of the phalanx can herniate. *(B)* Reduction is by traction and slight flexion, with immobilization in slight flexion for at least three weeks followed by active exercise.

(Fig. 124). Open reduction and surgical capsular repair are necessary.

The fifth carpometacarpal joint is also a saddle joint and resembles the thumb metacarpophalangeal joint. Open reduction is usually necessary in a dislocation of the fifth metacarpophalangeal joint, with a wire inserted to maintain the reduction. Degenerative changes ultimately occur following dislocation of this joint; these changes impair the cupping of the hand, thus preventing the formation of a good grip.

Carpal bone dislocations are common. A fall upon the dorsiflexed hand can dislocate the lunate bone in a palmar direction, causing it to protrude between the capitate and the radius into the carpal tunnel (see Figs. 14

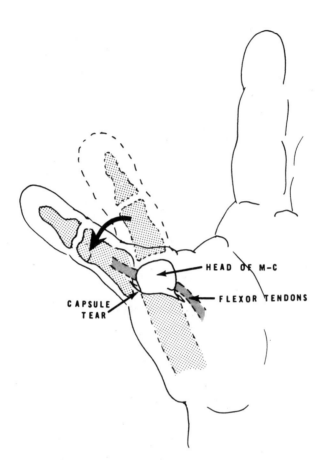

FIGURE 124. Dislocation of metacarpophalangeal joint of the thumb. The phalanx displaces backwards, tearing the capsule. The head of the metacarpal protrudes through the capsule tear and gets buttonholed in the tear and by the flexor tendon passing behind the head.

and 17). The flexor tendons and the median nerve are compressed, causing swelling of the palmar area and limited finger flexion. Median nerve compression or carpal tunnel syndrome may result (Fig. 125). Reduction can be achieved by direct pressure upon the palmar aspect of the lunate with simultaneous traction to the thumb and fingers. Healing then should be permitted with a cast.

RHEUMATOID ARTHRITIS

Rheumatoid arthritis is a systemic autoimmune disease with an unknown causative agent. Susceptibility to the disease appears to be an

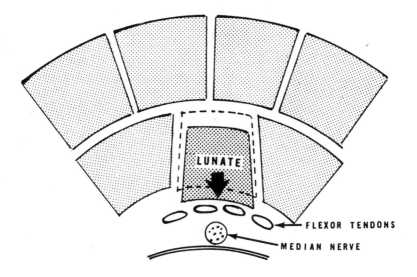

FIGURE 125. Dislocation of the lunate carpal bone. All the carpal bones by their shape, except for the lunate, dislocate dorsally. From a fall upon the dorsiflexed hand, the lunate dislocates in a palmar direction, causing swelling on the volar surface of the wrist and compression of the flexor tendons of the fingers and the median nerve.

inherited trait in which there is a histocompatibility of complex MHC in chromosome 6 involving HLS.

The disease target is primarily the synovium of joints and tendons, with secondary involvement of the periarticular tissues, muscles, and blood vessels. The synovium involved with leukocytes creates an antigen-antibody reaction forming a large molecular weight anti-immunologic globulin (IgM), otherwise termed a "rheumatoid factor," which can be isolated from the serum (Fig. 126).

The diseased cartilage and synovium phagocytes release lysozymes that in turn further damage the cartilage. Although the disease process is most often located in the synovium of the joints and tendons, other tissues are involved: the cartilage, subchondral bone, and intrinsic muscles.

Three alterations involve the synovium:

1. The synovial lining cells proliferate (see Fig. 126), thus encroaching upon the content of the joint.
2. The deep layers of the synovial membrane are infiltrated with monocytes and plasma cells.
3. There results an effusion of fluid into the synovial cavity. This fluid contains polymorphonuclear leukocytes and rheumatoid factor (see Fig. 126), altering the internal articular pressure and mechanics.

147

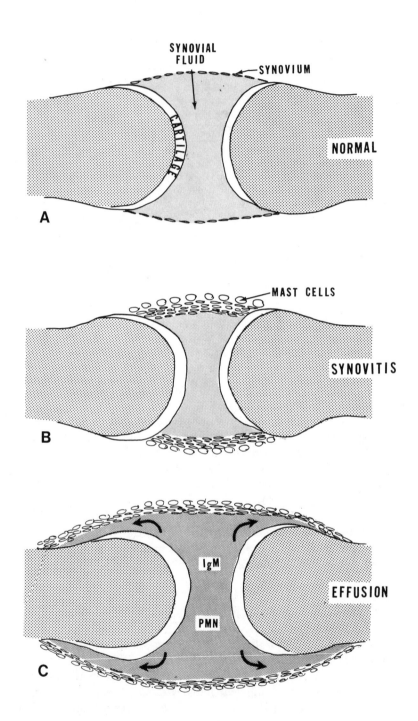

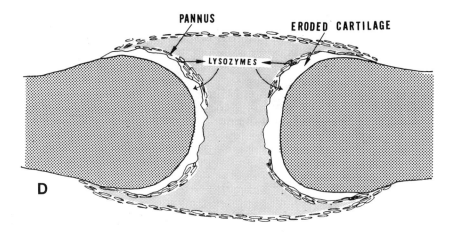

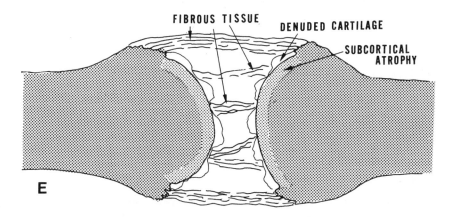

Figure 126. Progressive changes of joints in rheumatoid arthritis. (A) The normal joint with cartilage at ends of both component bones, capsule, synovial fluid, and synovium. (B) In early synovitis, mast cells appear with proliferation of synovium, leading to an increase and change in synovial fluid. (C) With an increase of effusion (synovial fluid), there is an increase in polymorphonuclear (PMN) cells and rheumatoid factor IgM. (D) The synovium gradually covers the cartilage (forming a pannus). The inflamed synovium secretes lysosomes and lysozymes that erode the cartilage. (E) The final stage may be development of fibrous tissue that connects the two denuded cartilaginous surfaces and causes a fibrous fixed joint.

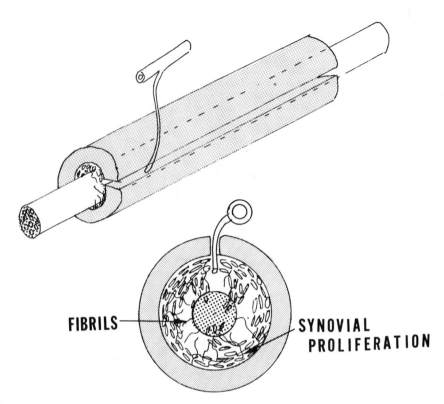

FIBRILS — — SYNOVIAL
PROLIFERATION

FIGURE 127. Tendonitis. Upper figure depicts a schematic tendon sheath with its two layers (see Fig. 30). In synovitis, there is an invasion of the inflamed synovium and microfibrils of connective tissue that compresses the tendon and adheres to it.

This process results in the following conditions:

a. Increase in joint pressure.
b. Stretching and thinning of the fibrous elements of the capsule.
c. Loosening of the bony attachment of these capsular tissues.
d. Interference with nutrition of the capsule, cartilage, and synovium.

As the capsule, ligaments, and all periarticular tissues become thinned, stretched, weakened, and even detached, joint instability increases. The synovium forms into a pannus that covers the cartilage. This occludes the synovial cartilage barrier and denies the cartilage its nutrition. The pannus forms into granulous fibrous tissue. Proteolytic enzymes formed from the pannus and the denuded cartilage further denude the cartilage. This nuded area becomes a site of fibrocartilagenous tissue that invades the

TABLE 1. Comparison of rheumatoid and osteoarthrotic hands

	Rheumatoid	Osteoarthrosis
Joint involvement	Middle row and metacarpophalangeal	Distal row
Wrist involvement	Usual	Rare if ever
Tenderness	Usual	Rare or minimal
Swelling	Soft of capsule and periarticular	Hand bony

joint space and attaches to the contiguous opposing denuded cartilage. In the early stages, the elongation of the capsule—with its thinning and weakening from distention—allows hypermobility of the joint, this then can lead to subluxation and even dislocation.

When fibrous organization intervenes, the joint becomes stiff and eventually ankyloses as the cartilage becomes softened and denuded, and the subcortical bone atrophies. Centrally, this softened bone can compress, microscopically fracture, or erode. At the joint margins, the cortex erodes and permits avulsion of the attached tendons and capsule.

Tenosynovitis

Tenosynovitis is usually associated with rheumatoid joint synovitis. The extrinsic tendons of the hand and fingers are involved in about two thirds of rheumatoid hands.[1] The proliferating synovitis fills the entire sheath and adheres to and enters the tendon. The most prevalent site of tendon involvement is within the sheaths (Fig. 127). This involves the extensor tendons at the wrist level under the extensor retinaculum (see Fig. 39). As the flexor tendons are sheathed through a greater portion of their length, they may be involved at many sites. The index, long, or ring fingers flexors may involve the entire finger length (see Fig. 29), whereas the thumb and little fingers are susceptible from the proximal phalanx, to the wrist, to the distal phalanx. The five finger flexor tendons are susceptible at the volar tunnel area (Table 1).

Tendons may rupture, causing mechanical functional loss. The cause of rupture is due to vascular impairment, synovial, invasion, stretch, and mechanical stress at points of bony pressure or angulation.[2] The flexor tendons exert greater normal mechanical tension than the extensor tendons and are more resilient. The latter are more prone to rupture.

151

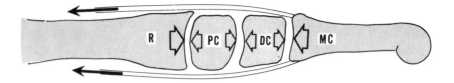

FIGURE 128. Carpal bone stability. With symmetrical dorsal and volar musculotendinous tension, the carpal bones are symmetrically compressed and maintain alignment and stability. Rheumatoid disease can cause imbalance of soft tissue with resultant carpal bone displacement (Fig. 130).

The Muscles of the Hands

The extrinsic muscles undergo vasculitis and inflammation. The intrinsic muscles are more vulnerable to concurrent joint and tendon synovitis. The intrinsic muscles undergo protective spasm to protect the inflamed joints, and by their action cause deformity, limitation, and pain. Prolonged intrinsic "spasm," albeit secondary, causes local ischemia and ultimately contracture.

Wrist

No tendons attach to the carpal bones (except the pisiform); however, in flexion, extension, and radial or ulnar movement of the hand, the carpal rows move on each other (See Figure 10 and discussion of the wrist in Chapter 1). The carpal bones are united by ligaments (see Figs. 7 and 8); therefore, when ligaments are attenuated by disease, these articulations are impaired. Abnormal pull or stresses by tendons indirectly influencing movement of the carpal bones can be detrimental (Fig. 128).

Joint inflammation and effusion of these carpal bones deform the capsuloligamentous tissues that normally support these joints. The volar ligaments, being stronger than the dorsal ligaments impose stresses upon the dorsal aspect of the joints. The ligament that unites the distal radial-ulnar articulation also undergoes attenuation with separation and instability of the articulation. The distal ulna migrates dorsally, causing the migration of the proximal row volarly and the distal row in the opposite direction (Fig. 129).

The extensor carpi ulnaris normally stabilizes the distal ulna by its passage over the dorsum of the styloid. If the tendon of the extensor carpi ulnaris is frayed, it can slip volarly and become a flexor, and simultaneously pull the fifth metacarpal volarly (Fig. 130).

A wrist (carpal) deviation has been documented as being a deforming factor of the rheumatoid hand. As a result of the powerful radial devia-

152

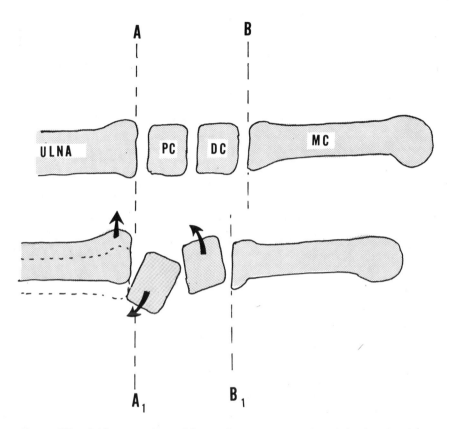

FIGURE 129.   Subluxation of carpal bones. Owing to asymmetry of the dorsal and volar musculotendinous pull, the imbalance allows carpal bones to subluxate.

tors (extensor carpi radialis longus, extensor carpi radialis brevis, and flexor carpi radialis) being unopposed by the ulnar deviation, the proximal carpal row migrates ulnarly.

The normal angle (Fig. 131) between the radius and the first metacarpal changes, causing radial deviation of the fingers (Fig. 131). The ulnar glide of the proximal carpal row, modified by the carpal ligamentous laxity and overpowering pull of the radial deviation muscles, changes the angle of the first metacarpal, and long tendon imbalance of the index finger then furthers the deformity. With the metacarpals radially deviated, the fingers assume an ulnar deviation.[3]

Thumb

There is a great flexibility of the carpometacarpal joint of the thumb. All ligamentous periarticular structures are strong, except on the radial

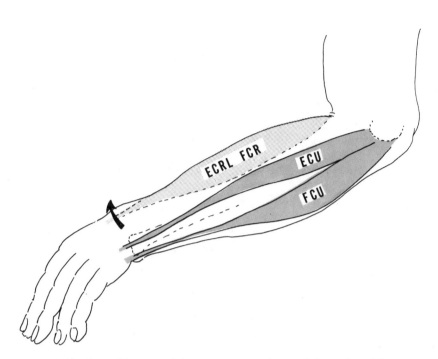

FIGURE 130.   Ulnar subluxation of the extensor carpi ulnaris. If the tendon of the extensor carpi ulnaris (ECU) becomes frayed, it can migrate volarly and become a flexor that ulnar-deviates the hand and pulls the fifth metacarpal volarly. A weakened ECU may allow overpull of the radial deviators: the extensor carpi radialis longus (ECRL), the extensor carpi radialis brevis, and flexor carpi radialis (FCR).

side. This weakness allows excessive adduction. In rheumatoid arthritis, with weakening these radial ligaments, the pull from spasm and contracture of the adductor pollicis causes an adduction and flexion deformity of the first metacarpal. Because of tenodesis action, the metacarpophalangeal joint hyperextends and the interphalangeal joint flexes.

In rheumatoid arthritis, the ring (fourth) and little (fifth) fingers undergo ankylosis at the metacarpophalangeal joint, frequently with 30 percent of cases undergoing excessive laxity. Because motion of these joints is largely rotational about a flexion and extension arc, this contributes to dysfunction of the hand.

Metacarpophalangeal Joints

Motions at these joints involve flexion, extension, abduction, adduction, and rotation (pronation-supination) (Fig. 132; see also Figs. 18 and 19). Radial deviation is associated with slight pronation and ulnar deviation with supination of the proximal phalanx.[4]

154

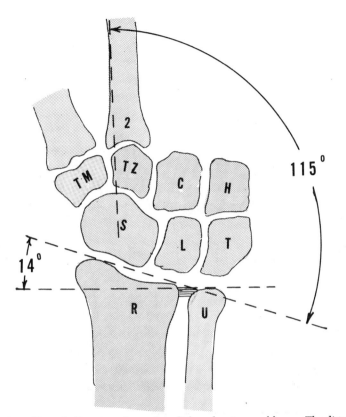

FIGURE 131.   Normal alignment of carpal, radial, and metacarpal bones. The distal surface of the radius and ulna usually has an ulnar facing of 14°. The second metacarpal "fixed" to the trapezoid (TZ) is in direct alignment to the radius at a 115° angulation to the distal radial ulnar facing.

The distal ends of the metacarpals (Fig. 133) vary in their angulation and in the length and strength of their collateral ligaments. Only the fourth (ring) finger is in direct alignment. The metacarpophalangeal joints offer no stability by virtue of their configuration. Support is provided essentially by the collateral ligaments and, to a degree, by the capsule. The palmar plates are suspended from the extensor tendons by the metacarpophalangeal component of the collateral ligament (Fig. 134; also see Fig. 19).

Ulnar Shift

About one third of patients with rheumatoid arthritis experience ulnar drift of the fingers. There are numerous factors that contribute to this deformity.

155

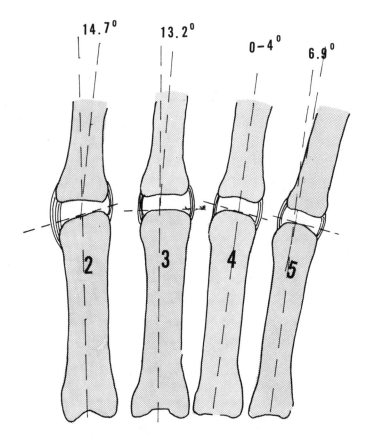

FIGURE 132. Normal inclination angles of proximal phalanx of metacarpophalangeal joints. The recorded angles are the range of abduction-adduction movements of the metacarpophalangeal joints. The differences in lengths of the collateral ligaments are also noted, as are their strengths. The metacarpal heads also have a radial facing in the second (2) and third (3) metacarpals and an ulnar facing in the fifth (5) metacarpal. There is *no* angulation of the fourth (4) metacarpal.

In the normal situation, there is a physiologic ulnar inclination in flexing the hand. This occurs at the metacarpophalangeal joint, especially in the index (second) and long (third) fingers.[5] The ulnar drift is probably related to *normal* joint structure with deformity brought about by external forces upon this normal joint.[6]

In paralysis of the intrinsic muscles (ulnar palsy, a collagen disease), the capsule and ligaments prevent ulnar drift (because of the intactness of the ligaments and capsules). Capsulectomy will not lead to significant ulnar drift if the intrinsic muscles remain intact, indicating that the muscles *can* offer joint stability. The ligaments offer the *most* support.

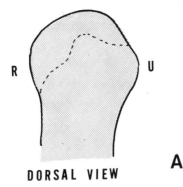

R   U

DORSAL VIEW

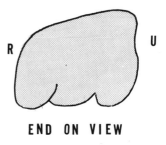

R   U

END ON VIEW

A

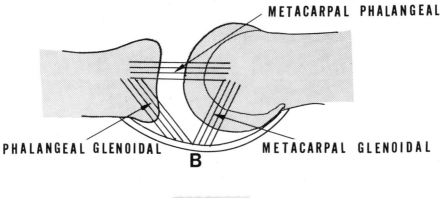

METACARPAL PHALANGEAL

PHALANGEAL GLENOIDAL   METACARPAL GLENOIDAL

B

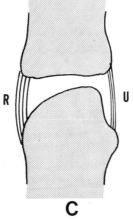

R   U

C

FIGURE 133. Metacarpal distal joint. *(A)* Normal configuration of the metacarpal head. *(B)* Normal ligamentous support of the metacarpophalangeal joint. *(C)* The radial ligament is thicker and attaches more distally; hence, it is longer than the ulnar ligament.

157

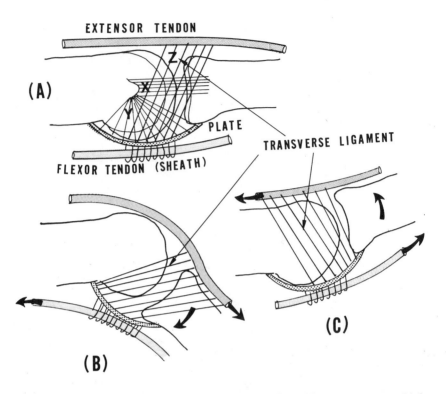

FIGURE 134.   Metacarpophalangeal ligaments. (A) The collateral ligaments comprise (x) the metacarpophalangeal ligament and (y) the metacarpoglenoidal component, which suspends the palmar plate and in turn the flexor tendons. The check ligament—transverse lamina (A) (B) (C)—connects the extensor tendons to the palmar plate and the flexor tendons (see Fig. 45) in neutral extension. The metacarpophalangeal ligaments prevent extension bowing; (B) in flexion, they are relatively relaxed; and (C) they extend the proximal phalanx.

Passive rotation (about the longitudinal axis) is limited to 15° by the capsule and, if the capsule is cut, to 25° if only the ligaments remain. Lateral and medial deviation of the metacarpophalangeal joint is controlled essentially by the metacarpophalangeal component of the ligament (see Fig. 133).

In power grips (see Fig. 37), there is adduction stress placed upon the fingers. The stronger radial collateral ligaments (over the ulnar) balance these forces on the intrinsic muscle (in the flexed posture) and do *not* contribute to extension or lateral movement, but act primarily as flexors.

With less than one third (30 percent) of rheumatoid arthritis patients developing ulnar deviation, the inflammatory process involves mainly the joint and periarticular tissue. In the early stages, voluntary contraction of the interossei can correct angulation. (The radial deviating interossei of

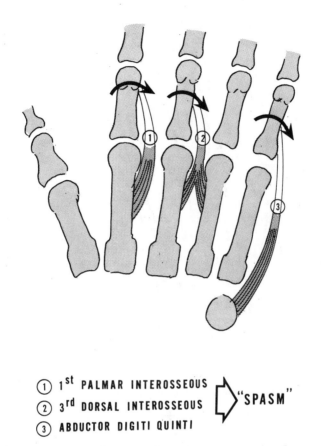

① 1ˢᵗ PALMAR INTEROSSEOUS
② 3ʳᵈ DORSAL INTEROSSEOUS ▷ "SPASM"
③ ABDUCTOR DIGITI QUINTI

FIGURE 135.   Ulnar drift caused by selective intrinsic muscle spasm, then contracture.

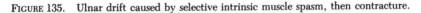

the index [second], long [third], and ring [fourth] fingers are stronger than the ulnar deviators.) This is true in extension, but as the fingers flex, the external control of the fingers by the intrinsic muscles decreases. It is in the flexed position of the rheumatoid hand that the lack of capsular and ligamentous support is *most* apparent.

In the normal hand, the radial ligaments resist ulnar deviation; and this resistance is even greater when the finger is flexed (in this position, they are made taut by being stretched over the tubercle) (see Fig. 18). In the two thirds of rheumatoid arthritis cases in which there is no ulnar drift, the collateral ligament must not be seriously weakened.

In summary, then, the primary breakdown in rheumatoid arthritis involves the collateral ligament, either by stretching, thinning, or detachment from its long attachment. If the intrinsic muscle *cannot* compensate, further deterioration occurs.

159

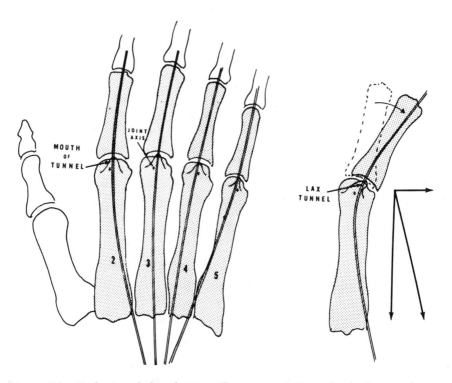

FIGURE 136. Mechanism of ulnar deviation (flexor concept). Normally, the flexor tendons enter the tunnel of the flexor pulley, which has a taut mouth. The tendons then veer in an ulnar direction. In the index (2) and middle (3) fingers, the tendon passes to the ulnar side of the joint axis. The tendons (4) and (5) pass radial to axis. Normally, the phalanges deviate ulnarly. In rheumatoid disease, the mouth of the tunnel becomes lax, permitting the flexor tendons to veer more ulnarly.

Selective intrinsic muscle contractures (Fig. 135) may cause ulnar drift.[7,8] Flexor tendon deviation force, by being freed of the restrictive fibrous flexor sheath, may cause ulnar deviation (Fig. 136). Extensor displacement is considered to be a sequela of and not a cause, but, once established, it maintains or aggravates ulnar deviation. Volar subluxation occurs (Fig. 137) because of laxity of the metacarpoglenoid ligament with "bowing" of the flexor tendon.

In rheumatoid arthritis, imbalanced musculotendinous pull against the collateral ligaments is considered responsible for ulnar deviation. The diseased intrinsic muscles are unable to compensate for the ligamentous instability. The radial collateral ligaments are elongated early in rheumatoid disease, permitting ulnar deviation. In this situation, the flexor and extensor apparatuses become active deformers (Fig. 138), causing further palmar luxation in an ulnar direction.

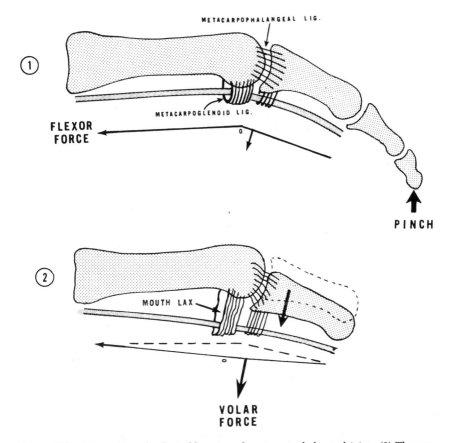

FIGURE 137. Mechanism of volar subluxation of metacarpophalangeal joint. *(1)* The normal pulley assembly fulcrums the flexor tendons during a forceful pinch. The normal mouth of the tunnel is the flexor pulley. *(2)* In rheumatoid arthritis, the tunnel and its mouth are frayed and elongated, permitting the flexor tendon to move volarly, thus causing the volar force to sublux the phalanx upon the metacarpal head. The metacarpophalangeal collateral ligaments are also relaxed, permitting this subluxation as well as ulnar deviation.

Ulnar deviation may be cosmetically unpleasant, but not necessarily functionally disabling. Most grip functions are retained if flexion is retained. The greatest functional loss is extension of the fingers as a result of dislocation of the extensor mechanism. If ulnar deviation is marked, however, the tip-to-tip grip of the thumb and index finger may be lost.

Ulnar deviation of the little finger cannot be ascribed to the same mechanism, since the flexor tendons bend in a radial direction at their tunnel mouths. One theory offered is that deformity occurs from the unopposed pull of the abductor digiti minimi. The hypothenar muscles attach to the ulnar side and are considered stronger than the palmar

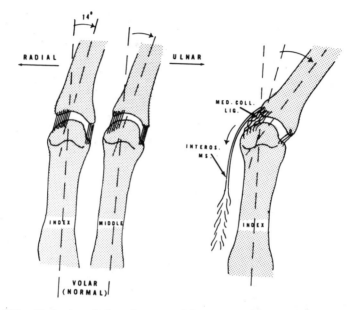

FIGURE 138. Mechanism of ulnar deviation of digits in rheumatoid arthritis. The normal hand finds ulnar deviation of the metacarpophalangeal of an average of 14°. This is most prevalent in the index and second middle fingers. In rheumatoid arthritis, the collateral ligaments, especially the radial side, weaken and lengthen. The intrinsic muscles are unable to compensate for this deviation and ulnar shift results.

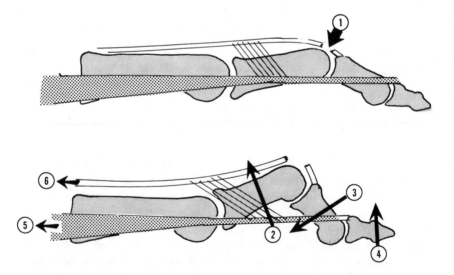

FIGURE 139. Boutonnière deformity. There is a stretch or tear *(1)* of the central extensor slip. The lateral bands migrate volarly *(2)* and flex the proximal interphalangeal joints *(3)*. The distal phalanx extends *(4)* and the intrinsics *(5)* and extensors *(6)* migrate proximally.

162

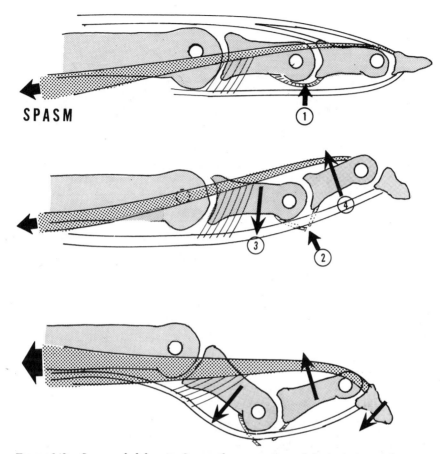

SPASM

FIGURE 140. Swan neck deformity. Spasm, then contracture of the intrinsic muscles causes hyperextension (4) of the middle phalanx. The volar pouch synovitis causes laxity (1) of the proximal interphalangeal joint with ultimate disruption (2). As the intrinsics move dorsal to the axis of rotation, the proximal phalanx flexes (3). Traction, resulting from tenodesis action upon the distal phalanx, causes the distal phalanx to flex.

interossei and lumbricals on the radial side. Currently, the exact mechanism of ulnar deviation of the little finger is conjectural.

Proximal Interphalangeal Joints

These joints normally flex or extend, but do not hyperextend or laterally (medially) deviate. The palmar plates are restrictive and the metacarpophalangeal and metacarpoglenoid ligaments are reinforced by the retinacular ligaments that connect the extensor mechanism to the flexor tendon sheath (see Fig. 134). The proximal interphalangeal joint is fre-

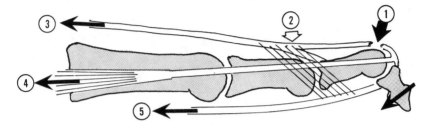

FIGURE 141. Mallet finger. A rupture or tear of the extensor tendon *(1)* primal to the insertion of the lateral bands *(2)* upon the proximal aspect of the distal phalanx allows horizontal proximal pull of the extendor tendon *(3)* upon the flexor digitorum profundus tendon *(5)*, thus flexing the distal phalanx.

quently involved in rheumatoid arthritis and, depending on which tissues become involved, decides whether a boutonnière deformity (Fig. 139) or a swan neck (Fig. 140) results.

BOUTONNIÈRE DEFORMITY. Disease of the tendons and periarticular tissues about the proximal interphalangeal joints may result in boutonnière deformity. Because of thinning of the central slip of the extensor tendon, the lateral bands of the extensor mechanism dislocate to the flexor side of

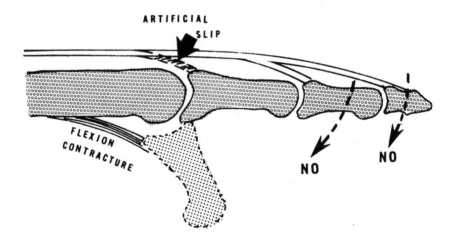

FIGURE 142. Surgical treatment of the metacarpophalangeal flexion deformity. The construction of an artificial slip to the proximal phalanx to assist extension also impairs flexion of the two distal digits. The flexion contracture is one of the disabling aspects of rheumatoid arthritis. If the extensor is anchored with fingers flexed (the proximal and distal interphalangeal joints), all long extensor action must be done by the intrinsics, which must be normal in insertion as well as innervation. This normalcy can hardly be expected in rheumatoid arthritis.

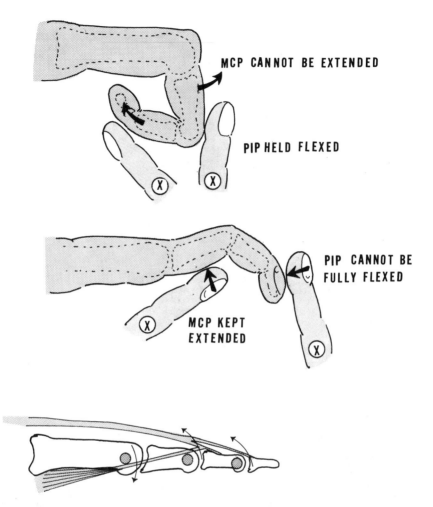

MCP CANNOT BE EXTENDED

PIP HELD FLEXED

PIP CANNOT BE FULLY FLEXED

MCP KEPT EXTENDED

FIGURE 143. Spasm of intrinsics. The metacarpophalangeal joint becomes flexed as does the proximal interphalangeal joint. If the metacarpophalangeal joint is passively extended, the interphalangeal joints cannot be flexed fully. Bottom illustration depicts the normal attachments and action upon the finger joints.

the joint fulcrum. This causes a flexion deformity of the proximal interphalangeal joint and hyperextension of the distal joint.

This deformity is difficult to treat. No functional splint is effective. Only a rigid splint can maintain correction that may have been gained manually. Surgical intervention is unsatisfactory because it frequently consists of severing the extensor tendon proximal to distal phalanx (which causes a mallet finger, Fig. 141) and reattaching the extensor tendon more proximally (Fig. 142).

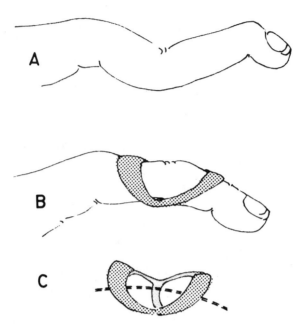

FIGURE 144.   Splint for swan neck deformity. Before contracture or subluxation occurs, the swan neck deformity *(A)* can be held or minimized by the simple splint shown in *C*. This splint limits hyperextension of the proximal interphalangeal joint and permits flexion of this joint *(B)*. (From Licht, S., ed.: Arthritis and Physical Medicine. Elizabeth Licht, Publisher, New Haven, 1969, with permission.)

SWAN NECK DEFORMITY. Spasm and contraction of the intrinsic muscles can cause secondary changes as exemplified in swan neck deformity (see Fig. 140). The proximal interphalangeal joint goes into hyperextension resulting from dorsal subluxation of the extensor intrinsic mechanism (dorsal to the apex of the rotator of the proximal interphalangeal joint). In this condition, if the metacarpophalangeal joint is held passively in extension, the interphalangeal joint cannot flex (Fig. 143). Contracture of the intrinsic muscles extends the interphalangeal joint and prevents flexion of the distal joint.

Swan neck deformity occurs in 28 percent of rheumatoid arthritics.[9] The metacarpophalangeal joint subluxes volarly (see Fig. 140), owing to spasm (with ultimate contracture) of the intrinsic interossei muscles, and the proximal interphalangeal joint extends. Flexion of the proximal phalanx is blocked, and a flexion contracture of the metacarpophalangeal joint occurs. By this finger position, the intrinsics are shortened and are thus encouraged to contract. The transverse retinaculum allows dorsal migration of the lateral slips of the extensor mechanism (see Fig. 139).

Loss of passive flexion of metacarpophalangeal joint movement impairs function more than does ulnar deviation,[10] but loss of flexion occurs without ulnar deviation.

This deformity can be averted by splinting (Fig. 144) to prevent a limited hyperextension of the proximal interphalangeal joint if utilized before contracture is manifest. If the joint can be flexed, the splint, worn day and night, permits the palmar plates and collateral ligaments to take up the slack. This splint permits finger flexion and thus maintains the integrity of the flexor mechanism. Discussion of surgical repair of this deformity is beyond the scope of this book.

Though swan neck deformity is most frequently caused by rheumatoid disease of the intrinsic muscles, there are other causes which also create deforming balance between flexor and extensor forces: (1) Contracture of intrinsic muscles causing flexion of the metacarpophalangeal joints and secondary proximal interphalangeal joint hyperextension are found in cerebal palsy and parkinsonism. (2) Flexion contracture of the metacarpophalangeal joints or of the wrist can follow injury. (3) Weakness or overstretching of the long flexors causes stretch of the palmar glenoid ligament. (4) Ulnar nerve palsy can cause this deformity.

Deforming contractures and hand postures must be corrected or controlled or both. The diseased part must be rested, and disuse atrophy from excessively prolonged immobility must also be avoided. Prolonged immobility impairs the nutrition of cartilage and periarticular connective tissue as well as the viability of muscle.

Early immobilization permits the beginning of recovery and a reduction of pain. Active motion is indicated early, but a *full* range of motion may be neither indicated nor desired. It is considered better to have a painless though limited joint motion or even a joint ankylosed in a functional position than to have an extremely mobile joint that is painful, unstable, and functionally inadequate.

Surgical improvement of the structurally deformed rheumatoid hand has definite value. Synovectomy has already been mentioned, but this alone will not correct existing deformity and dysfunction. If ulnar deviation is pronounced, the extensor tendons can be transposed over the joint toward the radial side to minimize the ulnar pull. In ulnar deviation of the little finger, the abductor digiti minimi may be divided and the extensor digiti minimi transferred to the radial side of the joint.

Reconstructive procedures vary according to the structural deformity and consist of division or deflection of the deforming tendons or the contracted muscles. Prosthetic devices are still in the experimental stage but hold promise. Fusion may be indicated when a painfully disabling joint laxity cannot otherwise be corrected and the patient can accept immobility of the joint as demonstrated by preoperative splinting.

167

Thumb Joints

Normally, internal rotation of the thumb occurs and is necessary for approximation of the thumb to the fingers and to the palm, the thumb being a fixed digit of support. In a large percentage of patients with rheumatoid arthritis, this function is lost. What grip remains is that of adduction of the unrotated thumb (opposition), and this permits only a weak and clumsy grip. If the range of adduction is limited, even this grip is deficient.

Limited adduction of the thumb merely prevents the holding of large objects. Loss of flexion or extension of the thumb metacarpophalangeal joint causes little or no impairment. The extensor pollicis longus may be progressively frayed at the site[11] where it passes around Lister's tubercle to insert into the distal phalanx at the thumb. This is an area of tendon that normally has poor blood supply and thus is vulnerable.

Intrinsic Muscles

Weakness of the intrinsic muscles is difficult to evaluate. Spasm and contracture can be tested as shown (see Fig. 143). Because the function of the intrinsics is to flex the metacarpophalangeal joint and extend the proximal interphalangeal joint, their flexibility (elongation) can be tested by *passively* extending the metacarpophalangeal joint while keeping the proximal and distal interphalangeal joints flexed normally. The metacarpophalangeal joint can be extended to 180°. Any limitation indicates contracture of the intrinsic muscles. An alternate method of testing is to extend the metacarpophalangeal joint passively, then attempt (test) flexing the proximal and distal interphalangeal joints. Since the metacarpophalangeal joint is allowed to flex slightly, the distal joints should flex further. These tests presuppose normal joint range of motion.

Evaluation of Functional Impairment

Functional impairment of the rheumatoid hand can be attributed to the following forms of tendon disuse:

1. "Snapping" tendons.
2. Stenosis of the tendons resulting from tenosynovitis.
3. Rupture of the tendons.

Rheumatoid disease of the tendons may cause formation of nodules within the tendon. These nodules may weaken the tendon and result in rupture, or they may impair smooth passage within the sheath and result in snapping tendons, also termed "trigger fingers." This condition may be

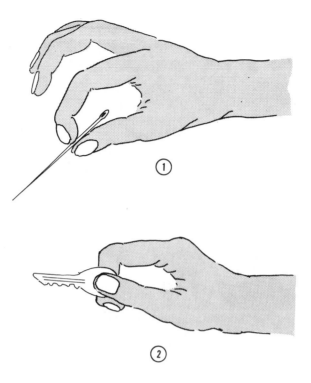

FIGURE 145.   Various grips of opposition. *(1)* Tip-to-tip opposition is functional and precise, requiring opposition of the thumb and rotation of the index finger in an ulnar direction (see Fig. 38). *(2)* The key grip requires adduction of the thumb and no rotation of the fingers.

treated by steroid injections into the sheath or by surgical decompression of the sheath. Excision of the nodule, if extensive, may weaken the tendon.

In evaluations of the impaired rheumatoid hand, all grips must be examined. Subsequently, each joint, tendon, and muscle must be examined individually to determine its impairment. Treatment, whether preventative or corrective, depends on this careful evaluation.

Impairment of any individual joint of any single finger does not indicate functional loss. Only by examination of the functioning hand in specific activities can the joint loss be evaluated.

There are four basic hand positions and activities that must be evaluated as follows:

1. Grip 1 is a tip-to-tip pinch of the index finger to the thumb (Fig. 145, top). To accomplish this, the thumb must be able to abduct and

169

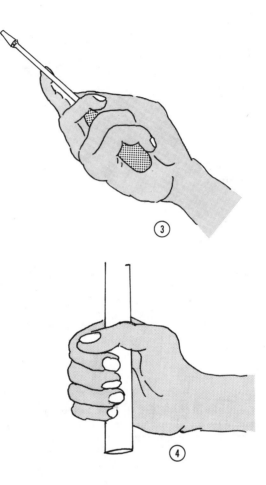

FIGURE 146.   Wrist-finger grips. The precision grip *(3)* requires ulnar deviation of the hand and fingers. The power grip *(4)* is used for such activities as hammering (see Fig. 47).

the finger must flex at the proximal interphalangeal joint. This is a precise grip used to pick up small objects.

2. Grip 2 (Fig. 145, bottom) is a more powerful grip (used in such actions as turning a key). For this grip, the thumb presses against the side of the index finger. For this movement, all joints involved must be stable and the intrinsic muscles (first dorsal interossei, adductor pollicis, and so forth) must be strong.

3. Grip 3 is used for grasping handled objects such as a knife, screwdriver, or scissors (Fig. 146, top). For this grip, there must be the firm grasp of grip 2 (thumb to index and middle finger), and the handle must be steadied by the ring and little fingers to the thenar

170

eminence. Loss of flexion of the ring and little fingers is a severe impairment of this important grip.

4. Grip 4 is a pistol or handle lift grip (Fig. 146, bottom). With this power grip, all fingers must flex enough to form a "hook" and the thumb must adduct to present as area against which to press.

In the early phase of rheumatoid arthritis, there is acute inflammation of the joints, tendons, and intrinsic muscles. The swollen joints can prevent adequate flexion, and spasm of the intrinsics limits motion. Upon subsidence of acute inflammation, the residual deformity causes the disability. This may be joint subluxation, joint contracture, intrinsic muscle contracture, or tendon disruption. The specific cause of the disability must be determined.

Loss of flexion as a rule is much more disabling than loss of extension. The specific joint impairment in relation to the desired grip must be specified; that is, the specific grip must be performed and the component individual finger contribution determined. For most functional grips, loss of flexion of the ring and little fingers is the most significant. The index and middle fingers function with the thumb, whereas the ring and little fingers stabilize the gripping of the object against the palm or thenar eminence.

The carpometacarpal joint of the ring and little fingers have a limited normal flexion range. However, if it is lost, this range presents a severe disability, since the finger cannot press against the thenar eminence; hence there is *no stabilizing grip.* Ankylosis of the joint in flexion is not disabling.

The metacarpophalangeal joints normally flex to 90°. A few degrees of loss in the ring and little fingers can cause significant functional impairment. Loss of flexion in the index and middle fingers is usually of less functional significance. Severe subluxation or ulnar deviation, or both, usually *does not* result in functional impairment.

The proximal interphalangeal joints normally flex to more than 90°. Minor loss is usually well tolerated. In the ring and little fingers, the critical flexion is 120°. Any flexion of less than 120° causes functional loss. Severe loss of flexion of all fingers impairs grip 4. Loss of flexion resulting from the hyperextension complex of swan neck deformity causes disability.

Loss of function resulting from loss of extension is not common unless the loss of extension is severe. Most normal extension occurs at the metacarpophalangeal and proximal interphalangeal joints, and loss of extension there merely prevents the hand from holding large objects. Loss of extension resulting from fixed (contracted) flexion must be severe to cause disability. Severe flexion deformities (allowing 160° or the normal 180°) are rare in the proximal interphalangeal joint.

171

Ulnar deviation, which is cosmetically ominous, is *not* a severe disability unless there is *also* loss of metacarpophalangeal flexion. The major loss usually is slight weakening of grip between the thumb and index finger.

Anterior subluxation or dislocation (palmar subluxation) occurs concurrently with ulnar deviation to a relative degree. These conditions are not a complication, but they usually develop together. Active forceful flexion of the fingers increases anterior subluxation *and* ulnar deviation. Subluxation of the extensor tendons occurs as a result of ulnar deviation, not as a cause. It occurs initially in the little finger and spreads to the middle finger. Once established, however, the extensor tendons aggravate ulnar deviation and extension of the fingers increases it.

OSTEOARTHRITIS

Degenerative arthritis, or osteoarthrosis, is a common affliction, known since antiquity and still eluding full understanding. Even without the serious portent of rheumatoid arthritis, it nevertheless causes pain, cosmetic deformity, and functional disability to the affected hand. Unfortunately, the label of "benign arthropathy of inevitable aging" has denied proper treatment to many patients.

Causes

Many factors seem to play a role in the disease. Genetic factors are dominant in women and recessive in men. Hormonal factors affecting the progression of the destruction and the metabolism of cartilage predisposed to ultimate degeneration are enhanced by enzyme activities. Unquestionably, mechanical factors are also pertinent.

The changes in the cartilage postulated to occur in this disease are noted in the superficial surface as a horizontal flaking (Fig. 147). This occurs probably to a greater degree when the cartilage has been predisposed to insult by genetic, hormonal, and metabolic enzymic influences enhancing the adverse effect of trauma. Cysts form in the tangential layers that open into the joint surface, causing rough craters. Enzymes such as hyaluronidase penetrate into the cartilage, causing loss of chondroitin, which changes the molecular composition of the matrix. Loss of cartilage elasticity results, synovial lubricants lose their viscosity, and further damage progresses until the destruction reaches the level of the subchondral bone. The subchondral bone successively fills in the denuded cartilage areas. Two incongruous opposing roughened surfaces with no interposed lubricant come to exist.

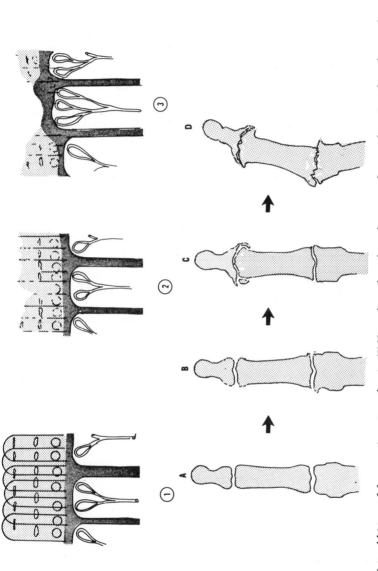

FIGURE 147. Natural history of degenerative osteoarthrosis. *(1)* Normal cartilage through stress undergoes alteration of cartilage surface. *(2)* Penetration of synovial hyaluronidase into cartilage causes degeneration of the matrix. Collagen fibers erode as does the cartilage. Subcondral vascularity increases, causing proliferation of bone into the denuded cartilage areas *(3)*. *A through D,* Typical x-ray results show changes from normal finger joints to early lipping of joint margins, with gradual formation of periarticular ossicles and severe erosion with subarticular cysts and the obliteration of the joint spaces.

173

Classification

Essentially, osteoarthritis can be classified into the following three types:

1. Primarily, distal interphalangeal involvement only. There may be some swelling, pain, and discomfort, with Herberden's nodes appearing. This type is probably a sign of aging, but it can also occur in young people; there is a familial tendency.
2. Generalized osteoarthritis, in which many joints in the body are involved. In the hand, the distal joints are involved most frequently, with the thumb carpometacarpal joint next most commonly affected.
3. Erosive osteoarthritis, which is destructive to the distal and proximal joints.

Signs and Symptoms

The signs and symptoms of osteoarthritis are stiffness, deformity, instability, crepitation, and usually pain or soreness. Since articular cartilage has no innervation, pain is *not* caused by softening or erosion of the articular cartilage. Pain arises from the *periarticular* tissues: the surrounding bone, tendons, muscles, ligaments, and joint synovium. The body's efforts to modify the stresses in the affected area result in the generation of more bone and cartilage. This remolding process induces more blood flow to the area. The swollen tissues and inflammation cause pain. Muscle spasm to "splint" the joint causes more pain, as does the inflamed synovium of the joint. This sequence explains the severity of the pain, swelling, and inflammation long before there is x-ray demonstration of the degenerative changes.

Often, after x-ray results reveal the osteoarthritis, congestion may subside and the pain may disappear. Heberden's nodes are frequently noted. The joints most frequently involved are the distal interphalangeal joints and the thumb carpometacarpal joint. Diagnosis is confirmed by x-ray examination.

Incidence

Degenerative joint disease is increasingly more common in older people, showing a marked increase in incidence during the sixth decade. In younger people, it appears predominantly in joints subjected to recurrent stress, such as the first carpometacarpal joints (trapeziometacarpal joint of the thumb).

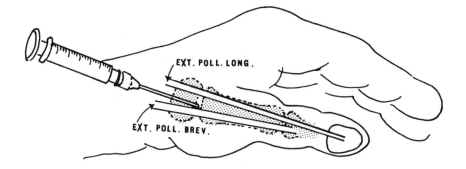

FIGURE 148. Treatment of arthritis of the trapeziometacarpal joint by steroid injection technique. The joint can be felt medial to the elevation of the base of the first metacarpal. Flexing the thumb into the palm opens the joint more. The needle is inserted just lateral to the extensor pollicis brevis within the confines of the snuff box formed by the two extensor pollicis tendons.

Osteoarthrosis of the carpometacarpal joint is almost as frequent in its occurrence as are Heberden's and Bauchard's nodes, which are the osteophytes seen in the distal and proximal interphalangeal joints, respectively.

Osteoarthrosis of the proximal thumb joint can occur without evidence of osteoarthrosis in any other joint. Clinically, there is tenderness by palpation, stiffness, pain, and, occasionally, swelling over the joint. Crepitation is noted on movement.

Grip is impaired as a result of painful abduction of the thumb and weakness, with atrophy of the thenar muscles. This condition is typically bilateral and more prevalent in women. Usually a history of trauma cannot be elicited. Diagnosis is confirmed by x-ray examination, but results from other laboratory tests are unrewarding.

Treatment

The acutely painful joint can be benefited by the local rest offered by splinting. Usually, two weeks of splinting affords relief. Intra-articular injection of an analgesic anesthetic agent with steroids also gives good respite from pain and inflammation (Fig. 148). This relief may be brief, but in many cases has significant duration to justify repeated injection. Salicylates are often beneficial, but the newer nonsteroidal drugs may be needed for relief. Heat in the form of warm water is beneficial and avoiding any movements that are painful is helpful.

Patients with osteoarthritis must be taught to live with their illness. The joints must be kept limber; therefore, in spite of discomfort, all involved joints must be moved frequently. Heat treatment preceding exer-

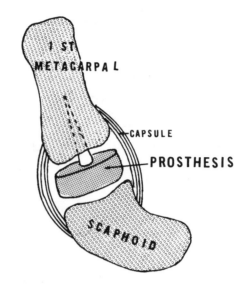

FIGURE 149.   Silicone prosthesis for trapezium replacement. This prosthesis requires an adequate capsule and thus must be done early after resection.

cises makes them more tolerable. The exercises are designed to prevent stiffness, and for this, heat is beneficial. Passive exercises (those administered to the patient) are rarely necessary, but active assistive exercises may be considered when a joint is becoming limited and contracted.

Surgery may be indicated for patients with painful disabling joints. Surgical candidates must be carefully selected. They must have full knowledge of the problem, full understanding of the procedure, and acceptance that the surgery will ameliorate but *not* restore normal function or appearance to the hand.

The most frequent procedure recommended is that of fusion of the involved joint, usually the distal interphalangeal joint. Fusion restores a functional position, removes undesirable cosmetic deformities, and relieves pain. Fusion may be performed by insertion of a *K*-wire after resection of the involved articular cartilage. The wire remains for approximately eight weeks, along with an external splint. The proximal joints must be moved.

Surgery may be considered for pain at the base of the thumb if conservative measures have failed to give relief. Prostheses are now available to retain movement and to relieve pain (Fig. 149). Although fusion of the base of the thumb (carpometacarpal joint) may provide a pain-free joint, this technique requires prolonged immobilization which may be unacceptable and can cause disuse atrophy or limitation of contiguous joints. A joint considered for fusion must be splinted preoperatively to allow the

176

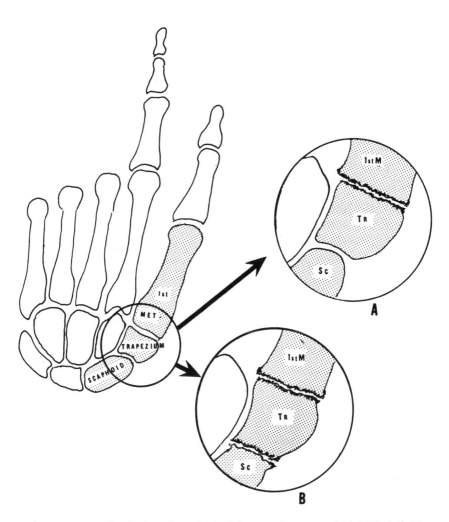

FIGURE 150. Surgical indications for arthritis of the trapeziometacarpal joint (A). Arthritis of the first carpometacarpal joint may require surgical intervention. These procedures consist of excision of the trapezium or fusion of the trapeziometacarpal joint. Excision of the trapezium gives relief of pain but carries danger of resultant weakness of grip. Arthrodesis gives relief of pain unless there is arthritic change in the trapezioscaphoid joint (B).

patient to experience the loss of movement and to accept that functional limitation.

Excision of the trapezius may relieve pain, but it shortens the thumb and decreases its strength (Fig. 150). Joints tend to become unstable after excision arthroplasty. The choice is a matter of the surgeon's experience and the patient's specific need.

177

Some degenerative changes in joints contiguous to the carpophalangeal joint of the thumb may cause pain and disability. The trapezioscaphoid joint may undergo degeneration, along with changes in the carpophalangeal joint of the thumb (see Fig. 150). These changes, themselves painful, may persist after successful treatment of the carpophalangeal joint.

When the trapezioscaphoid joint becomes inflamed, the flexor carpi radialis tendon, which passes near it, may also become inflamed. If, with the underlying joint inflammation, synovial fluid escapes into the tendon sheath, a ganglion may be formed. This palmar ganglion occurs infrequently, but, when present, its relationship to underlying degenerative joint disease can be verified by an arthrogram. The results will show that dye injected into the trapezioscaphoid joint seeps into the ganglion.

There are replacement prostheses for the proximal interphalangeal joints. If surgery is ultimately indicated, it should be performed by a qualified hand surgeon.

REFERENCES

1. Flatt, A. E.: The Care of the Rheumatoid Hand, ed. 2. C. V. Mosby, St. Louis, 1968.
2. Straub, L. R. and Wilson, E. H.: Spontaneous rupture of extensor tendons in the hand associated with rheumatoid arthritis. J. Bone Joint Surg. 38-A:1208, 1965.
3. Vaughan-Jackson, O. J.: Attrition ruptures of tendons as a factor in the production of deformities in the rheumatoid hand. Proc. R. Soc. Med. 52:132, 1959.
4. Rostler, O. C.: Histopathology of the intrinsic muscles of the hand in rheumatoid arthritis. Ann. Rheum. Dis. 8:42, 1949.
5. Brewerton, D. A.: Hand deformities in rheumatoid disease. Ann. Rheum. Dis. 16:183, 1957.
6. Shapiro, J. S.: A new factor in the etiology of ulnar drift. Clin. Orthop. 68:32, 1970.
7. Hakstian, R. W. and Tubiana, R.: Ulnar deviation of the fingers: The role of joint structure and function. J. Bone Joint Surg. 49-A:299, 1967.
8. Boyes, J. H.: The role of intrinsic muscles in rheumatoid deformities. The Rheumatoid Hand. L'exparision Scientific Francaise. Paris, 1969, p. 63.
9. Backhouse, K. M.: The mechanics of normal digital control in the hand and an analysis of the ulnar drift of rheumatoid arthritis. Annals of the Royal College of Surgeons, England 43:154, 1968.
10. Fearnley, G. R.: Ulnar deviation of fingers. Ann. Rheum. Dis. 10:126, 1951.
11. Swanson, A. B.: Disabling arthritis of the base of the thumb. J. Bone Joint Surg. 54-A:456, 1972.

BIBLIOGRAPHY

Bender, L. F.: Prevention of deformities through orthotics. J.A.M.A. 183:946, 1963.
Bennett, R.: Wrist and hand slip-on splints. In Licht, S. (ed.): Arthritis and Physical Medicine (Physical Medicine Library, Vol. 11). Elizabeth Licht, Publisher, New Haven, 1969, p. 482.
Carstam, N., Eiken, O., and Andren, L.: Osteoarthritis of the trapezioscaphoid joint. Acta Orthop. Scand. 39:354, 1968.

Duthie, J. J. R.: Evaluation of the patient with rheumatoid arthritis for corrective surgery. Archives of Physical Medicine 51:45, 1970.

Eaton, R. G. and Littler, W.: A study of the basal joint of the thumb: Treatment of its disabilities by fusion. J. Bone Joint Surg. 51-A:661, 1969.

Marmor, L.: Surgical management of arthritis. In Licht, S. (ed.).: Arthritis and Physical Medicine (Physical Medicine Library, Vol. 11). Elizabeth Licht, Publisher, New Haven, 1969, p. 237.

Moskowitz, R. W., Klein, L., and Mast, W. A.: Current concepts of degenerative joint disease (osteoarthritis). Bull. Rheum. Dis. 17:459, 1967.

Peter, J. B. and Marmor, L.: Osteoarthritis of the first carpometacarpal joint. California Medicine 109:116, 1968.

Shapiro, J. S.: Ulnar drift: Report of a related finding. Acta Orthop. Scand. 39:346, 1968.

Stillman, J. S.: The role of orthopedic surgery in the rheumatic diseases. Bull. Rheum. Dis. 20:568, 1969.

Smith, E. M., et al.: Dynamic ulnar-deviation splint. Arthritis Rheum. 7:467, 1964.

Smith, E. M., et al.: Role of the finger flexors in rheumatoid deformities of the metacarpophalangeal joints. Read in part for 18th Annual Meeting of the American Society for Surgery of the Hand, Miami Beach, Fl., Jan. 18, 1963.

Staub, L. R. and Chitranjan, S. R.: The wrist in rheumatoid arthritis. J. Bone Joint Surg. 51-A:1, 1969.

Wynn Parry, C. B.: Rehabilitation of the Hand. Butterworths, London, 1966.

Zancolli, E.: Structural and Dynamic Bases of Hand Surgery. J. B. Lippincott, Philadelphia, 1968.

179

CHAPTER 7

The Spastic Hand

UPPER MOTOR NEURON DISEASE

An upper motor neuron disease affecting the upper extremity poses difficult treatment problems. Upper motor neuron impairment in a child can result from prenatal and congenital insults such as anoxia, trauma, and vascular or infectious causes; in the adult, such impairment can follow trauma, vascular occlusions, neoplastic or degenerative disease, and cervical cord pathology. Each category varies in its severity, its progression, and its reversibility. The ultimate outcome depends on the cause, the patient's age, the secondary manifestations of disease, the patient's mentality, and the effectiveness of prompt specific treatment of the disease.

Recovery of hand function may be favorable in a patient with a small, benign, and favorably placed meningioma that is removed immediately upon discovery. Frequently, no treatment is needed for the hand after the lesion is removed. Evacuation of a subdural hematoma may also give favorable results. Hand involvement in multiple sclerosis may recover spectacularly as the disease undergoes spontaneous remission.

Upper motor neuron involvement of the upper extremity that persists after improvement of the primary cause poses the serious problem of whether or not further functional recovery is possible. It can be stated candidly that the amount of functional recovery attributed to current treatment is meager. Rehabilitation of the spastic hand is more philosophical than practical, and more psychologic than functional.

Wynn Parry[1] aptly states the problem of the adult hemiplegic with the following premise:

Anything more than a transient hemiplegia results in permanent paralysis of the intrinsics of the hand. Lumbrical and interosseous actions hardly ever return. There may be some coarse movement in the thumb, even some opposition, but controlled fine movements are not possible. All that can be expected of a hemiplegic hand is coarse grip and support.

This assertion does not negate all treatment efforts or designate all attempts to restore hand function as useless. Rather, it is a plea for realistic evaluation of the impairment, utilization of proven methods, and intelligent planning of treatment with concern for reasonable duration and frequency of treatment equated with sensible financial expenditure.

The problem requires long-term management with continuous physical therapy, proper splinting, and appropriate surgery. Treatment of the child is more promising because of adaptation and inherent neural pattern development processes. *Retraining* of the insulted adult nervous system, however, is more difficult. Objective evaluation and scientific documentation of proposed treatments and the resultant recovery are needed. Better knowledge of the natural history of the impairment's recovery is necessary, along with credited rather than glorified therapeutic concepts.

A rational evaluation of various modalities, standardization of techniques, and establishment of treatment frequency and duration must be undertaken. Recovery must be differentiated from maintenance of gained function, and a reasonable duration and intensity of treatment must be clarified.

This pessimistic prognosis concerning the adult hemiplegic is modified only slightly in the case of spastic hand in the child. Functional utilization of improper motions in daily activities makes children more educable but, in reality, improved functioning comes mostly through adaptation.

Following a cerebrovascular incident in the adult hemiplegic, the extremity becomes flaccid from the immediate shock, and gravity influences the position of the extremity. This flaccid stage may last for hours or weeks, although persistence of flaccidity for more than two weeks is a poor prognostic sign. Usually, there is a gradual onset of hypertonicity of the entire upper extremity. This is a release phenomenon from cortical control resulting in loss of voluntary movements, increase of muscle tone (spasticity), increase in tendon reflexes and clonus, loss of cutaneous reflexes, and slowness of remaining voluntary movement. Neurologic deficits cause the arm and hand to assume the spastic posture—pronated forearm, wrist flexed often in an ulnar direction, thumb in palm, fingers flexed at their metacarpophalangeal joints, and impaired extension of the digits.

Loss of *isolated* movements of the fingers and of all skilled motions of the hand is a severe impairment. There is loss of finger extension and wrist extension, with the hand assuming a clenched-fist attitude. The thumb is adducted and opposed into the palm and the elbow is usually flexed and the shoulder adducted. The patient is unable to initiate the opposite of any of these positions voluntarily. There is frequently a sensory loss. The finer, skilled movements usually suffer more than do the gross and less skilled movements. In essence, there is a predominance of uncontrolled flexor activity, and the balance between flexion and extension is rarely recovered.

Poor dorsiflexion of the involved wrist while making a clenched fist may be a subtle sign of residual spasticity in a partially recovered or initially unrecognized hemiplegia. Aged patients who suffer a cerebrovascular incident may experience the upper extremity assuming a catatonic posture during ambulation, yet be able to use it fairly well while sitting or standing. After a mild cerebrovascular incident with resultant spastic hemiparesis, clumsiness of the finer finger movements is noted more often than is a loss of strength.

During the early phase of hemiplegia, when flaccidity predominates, proper positioning of the entire extremity must be initiated with the assumption that ultimately spasticity will occur. During this flaccid stage, much damage may be done to the unprotected joint capsules of the shoulder, wrist, and fingers with resultant painful shoulder-hand syndrome, subluxation of joints, and excessive elongation of tendons and ligaments. Splints can be applied more easily at this phase than after the onset of hypertonicity. After the advent of spasticity, an uncontrolled, contracted posture leads to myostatic contracture, joint deformity, and muscular atrophy.

The position of the patient immediately after onset of hemiplegia is influenced by gravity, with the arm held close to the body and internally rotated, and the elbow and wrist flexed. Proper positioning must be established immediately (Fig. 151), preferably by the nursing service during acute hospitalization or by adequately trained home-treating personnel.

Pillows are placed under the arm to position the upper arm away from the body with the shoulder abducted to 90°. The elbow is positioned at 90° flexion with the hand elevated and with pillows ensuring partial external rotation. The wrist is maintained at slight extension by use of towels or splints (see Fig. 151) with the fingers kept slightly extended in a physiologic position and the thumb in partial opposition and abduction.

During this phase, *gentle* passive exercises should be performed daily with the objective of achieving the full range of movements of the shoulder and elbow, internal and external rotation of the arm, flexion-extension of the wrist, and full extension of the fingers and thumb.

During the acute phase, treatment consists of the prevention of contracture to facilitate any spontaneous recovery. Forceful passive exercises are to be avoided. The hemiplegic side also must be protected, but the uninvolved side is encouraged to assume *all* functions. From the outset,

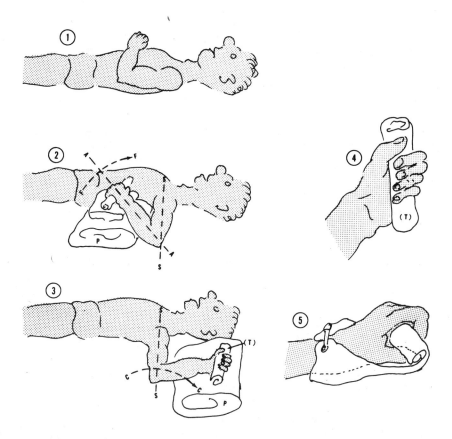

FIGURE 151. Arm, hand, and finger positioning during acute phase of hemiplegia. (1) The usual position of the arm—adducted to the body, elbow flexed, wrist and fingers flexed, and forearm pronated. (2) Pillows (P) are placed to abduct the arm to horizontal position (SS), forearm slightly externally rotated (FF), wrist extended as in 4 or 5. (3) When sufficiently mobile, the arm in the abducted position (SS) is externally rotated (CC) until resting upon the pillow. Wrist and fingers are kept in extension using a rolled face towel (T). (4) Rolled face towel is placed in the hemiplegic hand keeping the fingers slightly extended and the thumb abducted. (5) A towel folded and pinned as shown can keep the wrist extended and help keep the fingers from a clenched posture.

the concept must be accepted that ultimately the patient will perform all daily activities of self-care with the uninvolved extremity, and at best the involved extremity will be a gross helping arm and hand, but certainly not a painful and encumbering extremity. Any spontaneous recovery that occurs in the hemiplegic extremity will be considered a welcome addition.

Because the prognosis of functional recovery in the hemiplegic upper extremity is extremely guarded and unpredictable, it is realistic for the patient to begin immediately using the uninvolved side for all transfer

183

and self-care activities. Since the uninvolved side may not have been the dominant, skilled side, much training may be necessary. Effort in this direction should be emphasized. Independence is achieved more quickly with this realistic attitude, and the patient's psychologic acceptance of the impairment is enhanced.

In the mildly involved hand, treatment should stress bimanual activities, which should be done with the patient blindfolded to aid proprioceptive awareness. If a *mass* reflex motor response is invoked during an attempt to use a voluntary isolated motion, the patient should be guided to concentrate on separating the voluntary motion from the mass motion. Strengthening exercises of the weaker agonists should be performed. These usually consist of the opposition of the extensors to the hypertonic flexor muscles.

TREATMENT AND RECOVERY

Spontaneous Recovery

Spontaneous functional recovery from spasticity has not received significant study. Twitchell[2] observed that initial movement occurred in 6 to 33 days after stroke, predominantly in the distal musculature. Van Buskirk[3] found that functional recovery occurred in the first two months and *was spontaneous.* Bard and Hirschfeld,[4] in an attempt to prognosticate ultimate recovery, found that many patients achieved no recovery, but those who ultimately achieved full recovery had shown initial voluntary motion in the first month and almost all expected recovery within two weeks. It was their conclusion that the extent of recovery was evident within the first month, and maximum return of function within six months. Unfortunately, their studies rated gross motions and were graded according to range of motion, strength, and endurance—not functional recovery.

From these reports, there is good indication of the feasibility of intensive therapy for the first month after stroke, with treatment continuing thereafter only if significant practical gain is noted. Continuation of intensive therapy after one month with no recovery only tends to maintain the joint range of motion, helps to retrain the good side, and aids the psychologic outlook.

Exercise Therapy

Many concepts and techniques of neuromuscular re-education have been postulated on the premise that the central nervous system can be trained to regain voluntary control of the hemiparetic extremities. Many claims of functional improvement are attributed to each technique, but ultimate functional recovery cannot be attributed to a specific technique, as compared with natural spontaneous recovery or with generalized exercise. Many hours of tedious exercises have been employed, utilizing well-accepted neurophysiologic concepts and employing pathologic reflexes, but none has been objectively evaluated as to its practical, functional returns.

Peszczynski[5] rightfully questions the relationship between the concentrated learning of motor functions and the utilization of the substitution function. Do activities learned by intensive repetitive exercises ultimately become automatic unconscious movement? Does independent voluntary movement ultimately result from techniques employing mass reflex movements? In essence, can pathologic reflexes be converted therapeutically into unconscious coordinated motor skills? Extensive clinical experience with these techniques compels me to answer negatively.

The postulated progression of motor recovery in related developmental stages of cortical motor function, as described by Brunnstrom,[6] does not guarantee progression into the subsequent stage once a lower stage has been reached. Neuromuscular facilitation techniques using mass patterns, stretch reflexes, summation, and pathologic reflexes do not promise greater functional recovery than do simple active exercises. Motor activities are enhanced by sensory stimulation, such as cutaneous icing and brushing. These practices have the immediate result of reciprocal relaxation and enhanced motor activity. However, improvement does not persist, nor does it recur subsequently without more sensory stimulation.

Currently, neuromuscular re-education exercise techniques are experimentally attempting to apply neurophysiologic concepts clinically, as verified in the laboratory animal. These concepts merit further study, but they are not justified for clinical therapeutic use since they require extensive technical skill on the part of the therapist. Such skill is neither universally available nor necessarily desirable. Furthermore, these techniques require prolonged treatment, which is neither economically feasible nor justifiable, and they also give unwarranted optimism to the patients and their families.

Physical therapy exercises are nevertheless justified and desirable in treating the spastic hand. The weaker agonists, usually the extensors, should be strengthened. Repeated, gentle passive and active stretching of the spastic muscle groups should be performed daily. Brisk or forceful stretching of the spastic groups should be avoided, because it increases spasticity and is self-defeating.

Before any exercise or active therapy is undertaken, spasticity must be overcome or reduced. Removal or reduction of the spastic antagonist enhances voluntary function of the agonists.

Spasticity has been combated by use of neurophysiologic mechanisms such as the following:

185

1. Antagonistic relaxation of the spastic muscles, by attempting repeated and sustained contraction of the agonistic muscle groups. Since the agonists (prime movers) are often unable to be voluntarily contracted, pathologic reflexes are utilized in most therapeutic techniques.[6,7]
2. Slow, gradual sustained stretching of spastic muscle groups, which has been shown to release the spasticity and thus permit greater agonistic activity. Spasticity released by these methods is short-lived and not of prolonged functional value.

Medication

Pharmaceutical treatment of spasticity remains of limited value. Drugs specifically for spasticity, such as dantrolene sodium, have proved valuable in proper dosage. Drugs originally designated for their tranquilizing action (benzodiazepine, diazepam) have also evoked antagonistic action. Curare and curare-like drugs have received less enthusiastic support than originally, but still have limited value.

Modalities

Modalities continue to be a valuable adjunct to physical therapeutic approaches. *Heat* has its greatest value possibly when pain or soft tissue contracture impedes rehabilitation efforts; however, its value in overcoming or decreasing spasticity is limited. Ultrasound allegedly decreases nerve conduction time but has not been effective in decreasing spasticity.

Cold applied superficially and directly to the spastic muscle group appears to be the major beneficial modality. Total immergence into an ice bath has been advocated and claimed to be beneficial. The beneficial effect, however, manifests before the deep tissue temperature significantly decreases; thus, its effect is apparently upon the proprioceptors, spindle cells, or nerve fibers to the spastic muscles. Cold decreases the excitability of the muscle spindle and allows extrafusal elongation to proceed with greater facility. The type of spasticity determines whether ice will be of value through its spindle effect.[8] For example, spasticity due to hypersensitivity of the spindle cell responds, whereas spasticity due to alpha motor neuron activity does not. In addition, cold is brief in its beneficial effect upon spasticity and must be considered an adjunct to other therapeutic approaches.

Surgical and Chemical Techniques

Surgical intervention has been advocated in overcoming disabling spasticity. Tenotomies of spastic muscle tendons with total or partial release

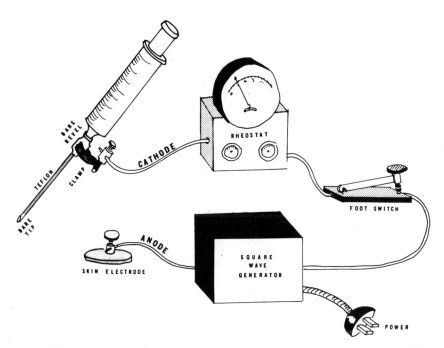

FIGURE 152. Procaine-phenol motor point injection apparatus. A syringe through which procaine or phenol solutions will be injected is connected to a 22-gauge 2- to 3-inch spinal needle that is coated with Teflon except for the bevel and the tip. A clamp connecting the cathode pole of a square wave generator is connected to circuit to modify the current, which is reduced to the lowest level that causes the muscle to contract. A foot switch permits the operator to manipulate the syringe freely. The circuit is completed by attaching a dispersing electrode to the same limb (anode).

have value.[9,10] In the shoulder, where spastic internal rotation and abduction present a major problem, tenotomy of the subscapularis muscle is an accepted beneficial procedure.[11] In a hand that presents severe flexion spasticity of the fingers, partial release of the flexor tendons has been advocated.[10]

Surgical or chemical rhizotomies or neurectomies that interrupt the motor *or* sensory nerve supply to spastic muscles are very valuable. Chemical neurectomies have been successfully performed with dilute phenol injected near the peripheral nerve or into the myoneural junction. This form of injection creates a motor paresis (via alpha motor neurons) that may last for 3 to 6 months, then usually facilitates a complete regeneration.[11,12]

During the paresis incurred from the phenol nerve blocks, the weaker agonist can be strengthened, contractures can be decreased, and functional training can be initiated. Pain may occur locally at the site of injection, and can lead to a reflex sympathetic dystrophy.

Chemical nerve blocks have not proven of great practical value in the upper extremity. Because the hand is so delicate in its functional mechanism, blocking of the hand flexors in the forearm at best releases the spastic flexors and permits greater extensor strength and range, but creates a better "helping" hand at best.

In an extremity with persistent, severe, and disabling spasticity, the spastic antagonist may be paralyzed or weakened by phenol nerve blocks, which then permit greater use of the otherwise overbalanced weaker agonists. Once the motor point of the spastic muscle is located by electrical stimulation through a skin electrode, the exact motor point is located more accurately by injection technique (Fig. 152).

The apparatus is a 22-gauge short-bevel spinal needle coated with Teflon throughout except at its very tip and at the bevel. Teflon is better suited than is plastic or collodion because it permits autoclaving for sterilization and penetrates the tissues more easily.

A standard square wave generator cathode pole with a foot switch in the circuit is connected to the needle bevel. The anode pole of the generator is attached to the same limb as a dispersing electrode. A rheostat within the circuit regulates the intensity of the current. Once the desired nerve is located by skin electrode, the specific site is localized by electrical current through the needle in which the minimum current causes the muscle to contract. Procaine solution, 0.2 to 2.0 percent, can be injected for relaxation from 1 to 2 hours. During this period, it is possible to differentiate spasticity from myostatic contracture. This duration also permits therapeutic evaluation of the strength of the agonists and the availability of voluntary activity after release of the antagonistic spasticity; it may also permit a brief period of active physical therapy during the absence of spasticity. The primary value of procaine is to determine the exact site of injection and to decide the feasibility of following procaine with dilute phenol solution (1 to 3 percent solution in distilled water), which may give a period of relaxation of three to six months.

Mathews and Rushworth[13] demonstrated the selective effect of dilute procaine upon the stretch reflex, and subsequent studies substantiated the selective effect of more dilute solutions upon the caliber of nerves. A highly dilute solution of procaine was considered to affect the gamma fibers, thus decreasing spasticity, but not to inhibit alpha fibers. Nerve transmission remained. More recent studies[14] have refuted the selectivity of phenol, which allegedly acts like procaine. Phenol affects *all*-sized nerve fibers, that cause wallerian degeneration. The selectivity appears in the larger axons where regeneration of the affected nerve is slower. The smaller axons undergo degeneration and regeneration faster.

Phenol nerve blocks are not without undesirable complications. Causalgic states may result or persistent areas of anesthesia may remain. Skin sloughs have been recorded. Mild pain in the area of injection with tissue induration is to be expected but usually subsides in a few days with no adverse effect.

One current concept of treatment for spasticity favors direct visualization of the nerve to be injected and advocates direct-vision chemoneurolysis as having fewer post-injection sequelae and better results. The availability of a skillful and interested surgeon may influence this decision, but electrode needle injection done skillfully also has its advantages.

Preventing Contracture

Prevention of contracture in the hemiplegic is of primary importance. Return of muscular function in a position of an extremity that is contracted is of limited value. Much of nonsurgical treatment has return of muscular function as its objective, with surgery being required when the program of treatment fails.

Connective tissue, which forms the periarticular tissues, is composed of three types of elements: (1) cellular (fibroblasts and mass cells), (2) fibrillar (collagen, reticulin, and elastin), and (3) ground substance. All these tissues occur in varying proportions depending upon the required function of that particular tissue site. Connective tissue undergoes constant change, depending upon external forces.[15]

Where free motion is required, collagen and reticulin form a loose mesh, sparsely attached: the greater the motion, the more distant are the sites of attachment. Where and when motion is restricted, collagen becomes denser and in sheets that attach at more frequent and shorter distances. The contracture is reorganization, *not* new or more collagen. The collagen fibers, however, *do* become shorter and thicker.

Connective tissue normally tends to contract unless it is combated by stretching forces. Without these stretching forces, contracture can occur in one week. With the addition of trauma, edema, and impaired circulation, it can occur in three days. The ability of collagen to elongate under moderate constant tension thus constitutes the basis for treatment. An acute, abrupt stretch is resisted by the tensile stretch resistance of the tissue. However, if traction is prolonged and constant, elongation will occur.

The modality of heat applied during prolonged stretching of contracture enhances the facility of elongation. In the spastic hemiplegic, local heat also relaxes spasticity as well. The type of heat applied varies with its availability, ease of application, and site of application. Hot moist packs (hydrocollator) or paraffin are accepted forms of modalities. In the clinic or hospital, ultrasound has the deepest penetration for the treatment of contracture.[15,16] Continuing stretch after the removal of the heat packs has proved beneficial.[17]

Once extensibility of connective tissue has been regained, it must be maintained. Where active muscular contraction is possible, this is relatively simple by the institution of *active* range-of-motion exercises. Where active contraction is not possible, then frequent passive stretch is indicated with splinting applied between the stretching sessions.

For the shoulder, the "bed" and "chair" positions must be ensured to maintain abduction to approximately horizontal position (90°) and the arm externally rotated. The elbow must alternate between full extension and 90° flexion. Because the tendency is for sustained (spastic) flexion, frequent extension must be passively or actively gained, then support splinted. Pronation of the forearm is predominant in the upper extremity synergies, and this must be neutralized and supination gained.

The hand tends to flex at the wrist, fingers with the thumb adducting into the palm. Towels and splints, both dynamic and static, must be evaluated[18] and specifically prescribed and applied. Each patient varies as to the type of problem, its severity and duration, spasticity and its degree, absence of sensation, and ease and availability of application. The choice of a mode of treatment must be determined and training must be provided for whoever administers the treatment (physical therapist, occupational therapist, nurse, family, or patient).

Pain Prevention

The hemiplegic upper extremity may present the problem of pain. This pain is predominantly in the shoulder and, to a slightly lesser degree, the hand and wrist. Other painful conditions of the shoulder, such as tendonitis and capsulitis, can coexist with hemiplegia.

In the shoulder, subluxation noted early in the flail stage is considered to be a common cause of pain.[19] There are numerous causes postulated from scapular downward rotation and functional scoliosis, to cuff involvement at the glenohumeral joint.

In the early flail stage, the use of a sling has general acceptance, but no complete physiologic or clinical benefit has been established. Recently, electrical stimulation of the supraspinatus, infraspinatus, and deltoid muscles has been claimed to be effective in prevention or correction of subluxation.[20]

Shoulder-Hand-Finger Syndrome

As the shoulder becomes spastic and the range of motion impaired, shoulder-hand-finger syndrome may develop (see Chapter 3). This condition is also known by such terms as minor dystrophy, causalgia, reflex sympathetic dystrophy, and so forth, and is characterized by these signs:

1. Limited shoulder range of motion (flail or spastic).
2. A swollen hand; initially edematous on the dorsum of the fingers, then ultimately the entire hand.
3. Vasomotor changes, vasospastic or vasodilatative.
4. Ultimate involvement of the elbow in many cases.
5. Progression through its stages sometimes resulting in a painless but "frozen" shoulder, and a stiff atrophic hand.
6. Osteoporosis.

In a few instances of the syndrome, a flail shoulder develops; in such cases, a neurologic vasomotor phenomenon appears to initiate the syndrome. In this type of case, as in the spastic or constricted shoulder, the hand becomes swollen and painful.

Impaired arteriovenous lymphatic circulation of the upper extremity is strongly considered to be a cause and sequence of the syndrome. As the shoulder becomes unable to move and to be elevated above cardiac level, the shoulder "pump" fails to mobilize venous and lymphatic fluid from the arm. As the hand fails to contract and relax, the hand pump fails to remove the venous and lymphatic fluid from the hand, and swelling occurs (see Fig. 93). The swelling occurs initially on the dorsa of the fingers (venous-lymphatic drainage, as in the dorsa of the fingers: arterial supply in the palmar aspect). As swelling occurs, it impedes the elongation of the extensor tendon, then ultimately the collateral ligaments (see Fig. 94). The edematous fluid is fibrinoid and protein in nature, and adds to contracture with further impaired motion.

Osteoporosis rapidly occurs, but its causes are not clearly understood. Undoubtedly, there is a disuse factor and also a vasomotor component. Pain may be present or absent. The vasomotor component may be absent;[21] when it is present, the entity is termed "reflex sympathetic dystrophy syndrome," or causalgia. This presents, in addition, the symptom of "burning pain" or hyperesthesia.

The duration of time between the occurrences of a stroke and the first symptoms of shoulder-hand-finger syndrome has been estimated as shown in Table 2.

Treatment is preferably preventative. Range of motion of the shoulder, wrist, and finger must be regained and maintained. If there are objective indications of vasomotor changes by cold, moist or warm redness, or a burning-like pain, stellate chemicals should be initiated early.

Massage, hot packs, whirlpool, and ice packs are usually poorly tolerated. Cool packs of 70° (21°C) are soothing.

Active range-of-motion exercises for the shoulder, hand, and fingers should be started immediately and should be done frequently. The part(s) that cannot be actively moved should be passively moved or actively assisted.

TABLE 2. Time between stroke and first
symptoms of shoulder-hand-finger syndrome

Months	Percentage of Patients
1	0
1–2	28
2–3	37
3–4	16
4–5	17
5–6	2

Intermittent vasopneumatic treatment may consist of a Jobst-type of vasocompression for the entire upper extremity or compressive centripetal wrapping of the finger with ¹/₈-inch soft braided nylon to remove or reduce the edema.[22,23]

Oral steroids in large doses for brief course have been found effective if not medically contraindicated.

If the frozen shoulder stage ensues—when shoulder (glenohumeral) pain decreases or disappears and range of motion, both active and passive is not possible—surgical release of the subscapularis may be advocated.[20] When a frozen shoulder has been ascertained to exist—when range of motion is markedly curtailed and an arthrogram reveals a severely constricted capsule (allowing 3 to 5 ml of fluid or dye)—"brisement" therapy may be beneficial.[24] This consists of injecting a large volume (40 ml) of dilute procaine hypochloride (Novocain) solution and triamcinolone under forceful manual pressure into the glenohumeral joint until the capsule tears and the arm can be passively abducted and externally rotated. This must be followed by active and passive range-of-motion exercises, with splinting to maintain the shoulder's newly acquired range of motion.

Bracing, when done with a specific rationale and indication, has value in preventing contracture and deformity. There are very few functional splints currently of value in the upper extremity.

The patient who is impaired largely from sensory deficit, or who fails to benefit from therapy because of sensory loss, may benefit from sensory retraining.[25,26]

Boyes[27] places great emphasis on contraindication of surgical intervention with spastic extremities, especially in children. These contraindications include the following:

1. Insufficient conservative treatment preceding surgical intervention.
2. Generalized muscular weakness.
3. Severe lack of voluntary control.

192

4. Presence of athetosis.
5. Sensory loss.
6. Severe emotional instability.
7. Low mentality.

In light of these contraindications, it can be categorically stated that most patients with cerebral palsy are not candidates for surgical intervention of the upper extremity. Rarely is an afflicted child a pure spastic or a pure athetoid. Rather, such a patient is a mixture of both, because of diffuse brain involvement. Along with the presence of spasticity, there is disorganization of neuromuscular activity. Antagonistic relaxation fails on attempting voluntary motion; the flexors thus contract simultaneously with the extensors, causing weakness and slowness of activity. Contraction of an agonistic muscle also initiates reflex activity of the opposing muscle groups. Surgery does not alter this abnormality.

Pronation of the forearm intensifies all other hand dysfunctions. The pronator teres and pronator quadratus muscles causing this posture may be contracted and must be released before any other hand-finger surgical intervention can be considered. The spastic wrist is usually in a flexed ulnar-deviated position. Extension is weak, if possible. The powerful flexor carpi ulnaris can be transferred around the ulnar border of the forearm and attached to the extensor carpi radialis to produce a strong wrist extension and to increase voluntary supination.

Wrist fusion is rarely indicated and must be preceded by prolonged plaster cast immobilization before surgery is advised. Fusion *is* indicated if transfer of both the flexor carpi ulnaris *and* flexor carpi radialis to the finger and thumb extensors places the wrist in marked and functionless extension.

The spastic flexor muscles of the fingers may be attenuated by partial flexor tenotomies that then render the extensors relatively strong and unopposed. Release of the sublimis tendons is all that is necessary, but the released tendons must be attached to the proximal interphalangeal joints to prevent hyperextension deformity of the proximal phalanx into a swan-neck deformity.

Before any surgery is contemplated, the procedure must be considered in relationship to the severity of the deformity, the ability and experience of the surgeon, the potential capacity of the remainder of the extremity, and the particular needs of the patient.

The deformity of the thumb in the spastic upper extremity is difficult to improve with bracing, splinting, and physical therapy, and causes marked restriction of function of the entire hand. Two deformities are usually present—thumb-in-palm attitude and the tightly adducted thumb. Both deformities prevent abduction and open-hand function as well as grasp and pinch motion. Spasticity of the adductor pollicis and the flexor pollicis longus are the major deforming forces.

Surgery consists of transferring the flexor carpi ulnaris to the extensor digitorum to decrease wrist ulnar flexion and to extend the fingers, transferring the flexor carpi radialis to the abductor pollicis longus, and releasing the adductor and flexion contractures of the thumb. The web space may require a Z-plasty. In severe deformity, an arthrodesis of the first metacarpophalangeal joint of the thumb may be desirable, after a prolonged evaluation of preoperative splinting or casting.

Summary

In summary, treatment of the spastic upper extremity does not promise much functional improvement with standard techniques of physical therapy, bracing, medications, or surgical interventions. A realistic program, however, must be undertaken in which maximum benefit is gained. The uninvolved extremity must be trained to its maximum for activities of daily function, with the involved side being trained to be as useful as possible as a helping hand. Ineffectual, prolonged physical therapy must be avoided since it places excessive financial burden on the family and the patient. Unwarranted enthusiasm may lead to ultimate disappointment and must be kept in check. Surgical procedures must be carefully evaluated to determine their possible benefit and to prevent any aggravation of further disability. Further research into therapeutic techniques, medications, operations, and modalities is necessary, but must be conducted objectively and scientifically, and so reported before new therapeutic recommendations are advocated.

REFERENCES

1. Wynn Parry, C. B.: Rehabilitation of the Hand. Butterworths, London, 1966.
2. Twitchell, T. E.: The restoration of motor function following hemiplegia in man. Brain 74:443, 1951.
3. Van Buskirk, C.: Return of motor function in hemiplegia. Neurology 4:919, 1954.
4. Bard, G. and Hirschberg, G. C.: Recovery of voluntary motion in upper extremity following hemiplegia. Archives of Physical Medicine 46:567, 1965.
5. Peszczynski, M.: Rehabilitation of the adult hemiplegic. In Mukherjee, S. R. (ed.): Locomotor System, Fourth Annual Volume of Physiology and Experimental Medical Sciences. The Physiological Society of India, Calcutta, 1962–63.
6. Brunnstrom, S.: Clinical Kinesiology, ed. 3. F. A. Davis, Philadelphia, 1972.
7. Rood, M.: Neurophysiological reactions as a basis for physical therapy. Physical Therapy Review 34:444, 1954.
8. Mossman, P. L.: A Problem Oriented Approach to Stroke Rehabilitation. Charles C Thomas, Springfield, Ill., 1976, p. 49.
9. Mooney, V., Perry, J., and Nickel, V. L.: Surgical and nonsurgical orthopedic care of stroke. J. Bone Joint Surg. 49-A:989, 1967.

10. Treanor, W. J. and Reifenstein, G. H.: Potential reversibility of the hemiplegic posture. Am. J. Cardiol. 7:370, 1961.
11. Mooney, V., Frykman, G., and McLamb, J.: Current status of intraneural phenol injections. Clin. Orthop. 63:122, 1969.
12. Halpern, D. and Meelhauysen, F. E.: Phenol motor point block in the management of muscular hypertonia. Archives of Physical Medicine 47:659, 1966.
13. Mathews, P. B. C. and Rushworth, G.: The selective effect of procaine on the stretch reflex and tendon jerk of soleus muscle when applied to its nerve. J. Physiol. 135:245, 1957.
14. Khalili, A. A. and Betts, H. B.: Management of Spasticity with Phenol Nerve Blocks. Final Report, R.D. 2529-14, Dept. H.E.W., Social and Rehabilitation Service, Washington, D.C., Dec. 1970.
15. Kottke, F. J. and Ptak, R. A.: The rationale for prolonged stretching for correction of shortening of connective tissues. Archives of Physical Medicine 47:345, 1966.
16. Gersten, J. W.: Effects of ultrasound on tendon extensibility. Am. J. Phys. Med. 34:362, 1955.
17. Krusen, F., Kottke, F., and Ellwood, P. E. (eds.): Handbook of Physical Medicine and Rehabilitation. W. B. Saunders, Philadelphia, 1965.
18. Kamewetz, H. L.: Massage manipulation and traction. In Licht, S. (ed.): Arthritis and Physical Medicine, vol. 11. Elizabeth Licht Publisher, New Haven, 1969, p. 405.
19. Cailliet, R.: The Shoulder in Hemiplegia. F. A. Davis, Philadelphia, 1980.
20. Lehmann, J. F., et al.: Effect of therapeutic temperatures on tendon extensibility. Archives of Physical Medicine 51:481, 1970.
21. Benton, L. A., et al.: Functional Electrical Stimulation: A Practical Clinical Guide. Rancho Los Amigos, Downey, Calif. 1980. Nat. Inst. Handicapped Research, Grant No. 23P-55442/9-08.
22. Moberg, E.: The shoulder-hand-finger syndrome as a whole. Surg. Clin. North Am. 40:367, 1960.
23. Cain, H.D. and Liebgold, H. B.: Compressive centripetal wrapping technic for reduction of edema. Archives of Physical Medicine 48:420, 1967.
24. Caldwell, C. B., Wilson, D. J., and Brown R. M.: Evaluation and treatment of the upper extremity in the hemiplegic stroke patient. Clin. Orthop. 63:69, 1969.
25. Simon, W. H.: Soft tissue disorders of the shoulder. Orthop. Clin. North Am. 6:52, 1975.
26. Goldman, H.: Improvement of double simultaneous stimulation perception in hemiplegia patients. Archives of Physical Medicine 47:681, 1966.
27. Boyes, J. H.: Bunnell's Surgery of the Hand, ed. 4. J. B. Lippincott, Philadelphia, 1964.

BIBLIOGRAPHY

American Heart Association, Inc.: Do It Yourself Again: Self-Help Devices for the Stroke Patient. New York, 1965.
Burkel, W. E. and McPhee, M.: Effect of phenol injection into peripheral nerve of rat: Electron microscope studies. Archives of Physical Medicine 51:391, 1970.
Granit, R.: Receptors and Sensory Reception. Yale University Press, New Haven, 1955.
Halpern, D. and Meelhuysen, F. E.: Duration of relaxation after intramuscular neurolysis with phenol. J.A.M.A. 200:1152, 1967.
Hartviksen, K.: Ice therapy in spasticity. Acta Neurol. Scand. 38:79, 1962.
Inglis, A. E., Cooper, W., and Bruton, W.: Surgical correction of thumb deformities in spastic paralysis. J. Bone Joint Surg. 52-A:253, 1970.

195

Kenny Rehabilitation: A Handbook of Rehabilitative Nursing Techniques in Hemiplegia. Kenny Rehabilitation, Minneapolis, 1964.

Khalili, A. A. and Benton, J. G.: A physiologic approach to the evaluation and the management of spasticity with procaine and phenol nerve block. Clin. Orthop. 47:97, 1966.

Knott, M. and Voss, D. E.: Proprioceptive Neuromuscular Facilitation, ed. 2. Harper & Row, New York, 1968.

Mooney, V., Perry, J., and Nickel, V.: Surgical and non-surgical orthopedic care of stroke. J. Bone Joint Surg. 49-A:989, 1967.

Redford, J. B., Gelewich, G., and Jiminez, J.: Simple Splints, Principles and Techniques. University of Alberta Hospitals, Alberta, Canada, 1969.

Reynolds, G., et al.: Preliminary report on neuromuscular function testing of the upper extremity in adult hemiplegic patients. Archives of Physical Medicine 39:303, 1958.

Samilson, R. L. and Morris, J. M.: Surgical improvement of the cerebral-palsied upper limb. J. Bone Joint Surg. 46-A:1203, 1964.

Stamp, W. G.: Bracing in cerebral palsy. J. Bone Joint Surg. 44-A:1457, 1962.

Swanson, A. B.: Surgery of the hand in cerebral palsy and muscular origin release procedures. Surg. Clin. North Am. 48:1129, 1968.

Treanor, W. J. and Reifenstein, G. H.: Potential reversibility of the hemiplegic posture: Results of reconstructive surgical procedures. Am. J. Cardiol. 7:370, 1961.

Walshe, F.: Diseases of the Nervous System, ed. 10. E & S Livingstone, Edinburgh, 1963.

CHAPTER 8

Hand Burns

The burned hand requires special consideration. It must first be determined whether the patient has sustained a second- or third-degree burn. Some burns may be a combination of both.

SECOND- AND THIRD-DEGREE BURNS

Third-degree burns involve *full* thickness of the dermis. Once recognized, they require urgent surgical intervention to prevent infection and ultimate joint contracture. This contracture ("stiffness") is not considered to be caused by the burn itself, but by edema and fibrous protein synthesis that results from the required immobilization as healing occurs.

The cause of a burn is an indication of its potential severity. Wet heat penetrates more deeply than does dry heat and can be considered to cause a third-degree burn. An electric burn produces a heat five times greater than a thermal burn and also is considered a third-degree burn. This is also true of an open-flame burn. A chemical burn is usually a second-degree burn.

Determination of the skin circulation may determine whether a burn is of the second or third degree. Pressure (with a hemostat) upon the burned area that causes blanching, then reddening upon release of the pressure, indicates a first- or second-degree burn. If the skin does *not* blanch, it is probably a third-degree burn (there is *no* redness upon release of pressure).

Burned tissues of a third degree create carbon monoxide therein; the carbon monoxide fixes the hemoglobin, bringing a brilliant red hue to the area. The fixed hemoglobin on third-degree burned tissues does not disappear on compression; hence, there is *no* blanching (a very reliable sign).

Skin thickness, which can be palpated, indicates the degree of burn. A second-degree burned skin is usually thicker, whereas third-degree burns cause thinning. As the examining finger moves along the adjacent normal

197

skin, upon reaching the burned area, an *elevation* of the burned skin implies a second-degree burn, whereas a *depression* suggests a third-degree burn. *Loss of sensation* of a burned area is *not* a sensitive indication of degree of burn. All degrees of burns have impaired sensation.

TREATMENT

This chapter covers treatment specific to the burned hand and fingers, not the local or general care of burns.

Acute Phase

Management in the acute phase consists of pain control, wound healing, maintenance of range of motion, prevention of infection, and self-care. An exercise program is initiated within the first 48 to 72 hours and is carried out two to four times a day. All involved joints receive active or active-assistive exercise. Nonburned extremities are actively or actively-assistively exercised to prevent stasis, disuse, and psychological deterioration, and to promote self-care.

Hydrotherapy for wound care is usually begun immediately upon admission to a health care facility and continued when the patient receives an autograft or homograft. Hydrotherapy and exercises are resumed five days postgraft to and are applied to the grafted site and to the donor site. If porcine heterographs are used daily, hydrotherapy and exercise are used sooner.

Local (acute) wound care consists of using sterile sponge, mesh, or washcloth to each open area. A mild nonirritating soap (Dial or Ivory) may be used if it is necessary to remove film, exudate or previously applied topical agents. The best cleaning agent derives from the mechanical effect of copious amounts of plain water. Strong antiseptic soaps should *not* be used. Any agent used should be removed by copious rinsing.

The area then should be covered by a dry sterile mesh dressing. A course mesh dressing stimulates the growth of granulation tissue. A fine mesh dressing helps to flatten the areas of new granulation tissue. The mesh dressings (patches) are applied wet with sterile water and allowed to dry.

If dry dressings cause pain or excessive discomfort, wounds may be dressed with silver sulfadiazine or neomycin. Areas of excessive uncontrolled granulation tissue that do not respond to fine-mesh patches can be treated by one or two applications of silver nitrate.

Blisters that are intact are not susceptible to infection, however, once ruptured, they may become susceptible. Unless ruptured, the blisters should be left alone since usually they reabsorb. Upon resorption of the fluid, the skin (of the blister) wrinkles. This wrinkled skin can be removed easily. If the blister is large and covers a wide area containing copious amounts of fluid, it may *not* resolve. Such a blister may be drained prophylactically and the debris (epidermis) cleared away. The denuded area must then be aseptically treated. If a blister ruptures spontaneously, the epithelial debris should be removed aseptically.

A debrided second-degree burn usually heals with exposure as the only further treatment. A blood "clot" forms and seals the denuded area. Within 7 to 10 days, epithelium begins forming under the clot. Usually this is not a true blood-containing clot and can be easily disrupted; hence, the part must be immobilized to prevent disruption of the clot. However, this can be impractical and often undesirable.

An artificial clot is thus considered more desirable. Painting these areas with mercurochrome may hasten drying and crusting. A dry, fine-mesh gauze and bandage may be considered. Application of a mesh raises the risk of infection and must be applied with *utmost* asepsis; that is, the physician must use mask and gloves, the area must be cleaned thoroughly with surgical soap and sterile water, and careful debridement of excessive skin, blisters, and so forth must take place. Skin adjacent to the burned area must be treated with an antiseptic agent. The gauze applied to the burned area should *not* be impregnated with any medication, such as an antibiotic agent or vaseline. A dry sterile gauze left over the area for 7 to 10 days will allow epithelium to form over the burned area. Should infection intervene, the gauze is removed and continuous, warm, sterile saline and wet dressings should be applied until the wound is clean. Systemic antibiotics should be given.

As a rule, early surgery is being advocated for third-degree burns. Under local or general anesthesia, the burned skin is excised and replaced immediately with split-thickness skin grafts.

Physical management of the burned hand (by physical and occupational therapists assisting the physician) remains controversial as to its specific details. The hand must be maintained in elevation to decrease or resolve edema. The goal is to keep the skin or scar as soft, pliable, and flat as possible. This is accomplished by use of heat, lubrication, massage, and pressure with proper positioning and intermittent elevation while healing occurs and the skin matures.

Edema can be decreased by enclosing the hand in a gauze stockinet that encircles the wrist, hand, and fingers and extends sufficiently distal to be attached to an overhead apparatus. A Fiberglas splint may be applied over the stockinet base (Fig. 153).

Gentle, sustained stretching lengthens the bands of scar tissue and increases the joint range of motion. Massage after a paraffin application also maintains pliability. Deep massage of the subcutaneous tissue must avoid friction of the superficial layers that can cause blisters.

199

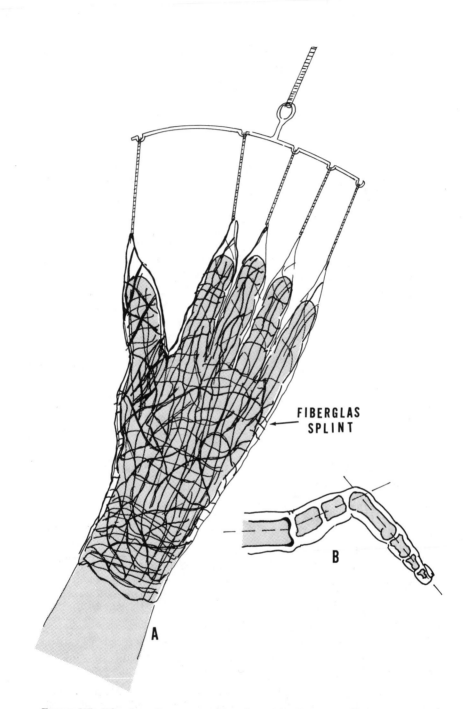

FIBERGLAS
SPLINT

A

B

FIGURE 153. Fiberglas splint over stockinet base (A). This splint holds the hand with the wrist in slight extension. The metacarpal joints are in slight flexion and the interphalangeal joints are in extension (B). The hand can be held elevated by an overhead traction.

Subacute Phase

Burn scars contract and have a tendency to become hypertrophic and to limit functioning of affected parts. Scarring, with its loss of elasticity, leads to decreased joint motion with resultant pain and dysfunction. Joint stiffness results from collagen synthesis and degradation with rapid remodeling within the joint capsules and collateral ligaments.[1] Thus, it is mandatory that joint mobility be maintained.

Joint mobility is dependent upon exercise in spite of the adverse effect of dryness and decreased elasticity of the scar tissue about or across joints.

Slow, sustained stretching is the most effective method of increasing and maintaining the length of scar tissue. Lubrication of the skin during exercise combats dryness. Heat enhances elongation and remodeling of connective tissue scarring, increases circulation, relieves pain, and relaxes muscle spasm. Heat increases and maintains the extensibility of collagen tissue both during its application and for some time afterward. This principle underlies the stretching procedures used during and after heat therapy.[2]

Hydrotherapy is sometimes advocated, but water temperature cannot be maintained or tolerated at a sufficiently high heat for a prolonged period of time. The patient may exercise more freely in the water, but prolonged submersion has a drying effect that ultimately decreases skin pliability.

Paraffin has been proven effective as a method for applying heat and simultaneous lubrication. However, paraffin should *not* be applied too early where open areas persist, during the "fragile blistering stage," or when scars are considered immature. The temperature of the paraffin must also be considered before its application and may be a contraindication if the *new* skin is too fragile or too hypersensitive to a temperature of 37 to 38°C (the temperature of liquid paraffin).

Paraffin is applied by equipment available in most physical therapy departments. Paraffin has a melting point of 34°C. Heavy-duty mineral oil is mixed with paraffin at a ratio of 2.5 ounces (75 grams) mineral oil to 1 pound (450 grams) paraffin. The temperature of the machine is then lowered to 33°C or slightly less.

The paraffin-oil is then applied (to the hand and fingers) by dipping the injured hand into the solution eight to ten times until a thick coating is obtained. A patient with limited finger flexion should make as tight a fist as possible before dipping. A small cone or cylinder may be placed in the hand and the patient is encouraged to "squeeze" before dipping. After being dipped, the hand is covered with a plastic wrap and is held in flexion by an ace bandage and is exercised, stretched, or massaged. The bandage must *not* be constrictive but merely supportive. Air must have access to the hand and the hand must be visible.

201

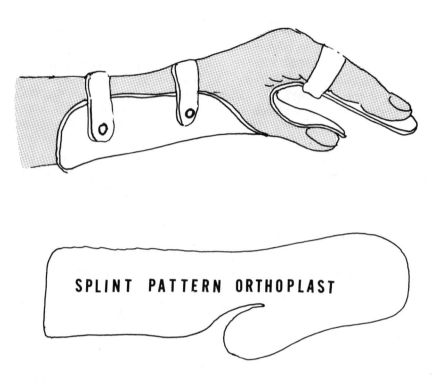

FIGURE 154. Isoplast isoprene splint. Models are made in several-size patterns for immediate application. The plastic is heated by hot water or heat gun, then cut and molded easily to the patient's hand. (Adapted from Willis, B.: The use of orthoplast isoprene splints in the treatment of the acutely burned child. Am. J. Occup. Ther. 23:57, 1969.)

During the posthealing stage, splinting, in addition to active and active-assistive exercises, is beneficial to decrease hypertrophic scarring and prevent deformity. Several questions must be asked before corrective splinting is applied:

1. Will the newly healed skin tolerate the stress?
2. Will the scar best be treated by constant pressure or by dynamic stretching?
3. Will the patient tolerate the orthotic device in regard to pain, discomfort, or cosmetic appearance?
4. Can the splint be accepted for the duration required?

Splints considered *conforming* are widely used in burn care. They are constructed from isoprene plastic. (Fig. 154). This material is treated until moldable, then applied (molded) directly to the body for maximum contact with the scar on the fibrous band. The splint produces hard, unyielding pressure that gradually softens, flattens, and remolds the contour of the part splinted. Conforming splints are of value when contracture develops over the volar (palmar) aspect of the hand, wrist, and elbow, or the the finger web spaces.

Serial splinting can be used to correct a contracture; this requires periodic evaluation with application with simultaneous active and active-assistive exercises. As a rule of splinting, stretch is provided for burns of the extensor surface of the hands, usually via rubber bands attached to the fingers from a wrist cock-up splint. Palmar burns respond best with constant hard pressure applied along the entire surface of the hand and fingers. If both surfaces are burned, a combination of palmar pressure and extensor traction is used.

The position of the hand-wrist and fingers deserves special consideration. The wrist must not be permitted to assume flexion from gravity. A slight degree of wrist flexion must be attained by a splint. This (wrist) splint, worn day and night, allows functional use of the hand and permits exercise. This extension of approximately 15° is desirable and allows wrist extension exercises above that degree of immobilization.

The metacarpophalangeal joints are so frequently involved in dorsal burns of the hand that they require special concern. These joints tend to contract and, if immobilized, become shortened *in extension*. The splint must therefore position the fingers at the metacarpophalangeal joint *in flexion*. This splint is maintained at night (along with elevation) and during the day between the periods of active-passive joint movement.

With the finger metacarpophalangeal joints flexed, the thumb web cannot be fully extended even though the thumb is abducted. During the day, this must be kept in mind and the thumb must be passively stretched frequently. If the thumb has been burned, it should be included into the splint that places the thumb under constant stretch. Full extension of the thumb metacarpophalangeal joint must be achieved repeatedly. With the fingers in slight flexion at the metacarpophalangeal joints, the interphalangeal joint must be kept extended. Daytime active flexion is instituted.

If the dorsum of the thumb is so severely burned as to threaten ultimate contracture and joint immobilization, the thumb must be kept immobilized in the flexed position of opposition by splint, either dynamic (preferably) or static. The thumb opposition splint attachment can be added to the hand splint, which slightly extends the wrist and flexes the metacarpophalangeal joint. Because the forces of the splint are in one direction, counterpressure or immobilization properties may have to be built into the splint.

The hand, wrist and fingers, in essence, must be splinted into a functional position in the advent of contracture, but must be kept as mobile as possible by active-passive exercises (see Fig. 84).

Because the elbow and shoulder must retain proper position and achieve range to place the hand in a functional position, careful observation and treatment are necessary to ensure this action.

In summary, treatment of the burned upper extremity presents an ongoing, constantly changing problem that requires frequent evaluation and modification of techniques and modalities, but always with the objective of maintaining functional position and action.

REFERENCES

1. Peacock, E. E., Madden, J. W., and Trier, W. C.: Some studies on the treatment of burned hands. Ann. Surg. 171:903, 1970.
2. Shull, J. R.: Heating modalities. South. Med. J. 61:621, 1968.

BIBLIOGRAPHY

Abramson, D. I., et al: Effect of paraffin bath and hot fomentations on local tissue temperatures. Archives of Physical Medicine 45:87, 1964.

Boswick, J. A., Jr.: Management of the burned hand. Orthop. Clin. North Am. 1:311, 1970.

Boswick, J. A.: Rehabilitation of the burned hand. Clin. Orthop. 104:162, 1974.

Gromley, J. K.: Rehabilitation of the burned hand. Archives of Physical Medicine 43:508, 1962.

Head, M. D. and Helms, P. A.: Paraffin and sustained stretching in the treatment of burn contractures. Burns 4:136, 1977.

Helm, P. A., et al: Burn rehabilitation—a team approach. Surg. Clin. North Am. 58:1263, 1978.

Huang, T. T., Larson, D. L., and Lewis, S. R.: Burned hands. Plast. Reconstr. Surg. 56:21, 1975.

Jaeger, D. L.: Maintenance of function of the burn patient. Phys. Ther. 52:627, 1972.

Koepke, G. H. The role of physical medicine in the treatment of burns. Surg. Clin. North Am. 50:1385, 1970.

Koepke, G. H., Feallock, B., and Feller, I.: Splinting of the severely burned hand. Am. J. Occup. Ther. 17:147, 1963.

Larsen, D. L. and Abston, S. Techniques for decreasing scar formation and contractures in the burned patient. J. Trauma 10:807, 1971.

Larson, D. L., et al.: Skeletal suspension and traction in the treatment of pain. Ann. Surg. 168:981, 1964.

Salisbury, R. E. and Palm, L.: Dynamic splinting for dorsal burns of the hand. Plast. Reconstr. Surg. 51:226, 1973.

Spinner, M., et al.: Impending ischemic contracture of the hand. Plast. Reconstr. Surg. 50:341, 1972.

Torres, J. Little finger splint. Am. J. Occup. Ther. 29:230, 1975.

Whitson, T. C., et al.: Management of the burned hand. J. Trauma 11:606, 1971.

Willis, B.: The use of orthoplast isoprene splints in the treatment of the acutely burned child: Preliminary report. Am. J. Occup. Ther. 23:57, 1969.

Willis, B.: A follow-up: The use of orthoplast isoprene splints in the treatment of the actuely burned child. Am. J. Occup. Ther. 24:187, 1970.

CHAPTER 9

Infections and Vascular Impairment of the Hand

INFECTIONS

Today, with the availability of newer broad-spectrum antibiotics and the ability to determine drug specificity for a given pathogenic organism, hand infections no longer create the havoc they once did. The infected hand usually responds favorably and rapidly to early recognition and treatment. A trivial injury, however, such as a small laceration or abrasion, may spread into the fascial sheaths, tendon sheaths, or lymphatics and present a serious problem before antibiotic therapy is instituted. As in most infections, proper care requires incision, drainage, and specific antibiotic medication.

Felon

A pyogenic infection in the terminal pulp space is called a felon (Fig. 155). Pain and swelling of the terminal digit block the circulation to that digit and may result in ultimate necrosis of the bone diaphysis. A felon demands prompt and adequate drainage, best executed in a bloodless field.

Between the bone and the skin, the pulp contains many vertical septa that form numerous compartments. These can be drained adequately only by incising *across* the columns. The incision must be made near the nail to avoid scar formation over sensitive tactile pad surfaces. Care must be exercised to avoid cutting the distal flexor tendon. If a sizable bone sequestrum has formed, it must be excised. Minor bone sequestra will regenerate if the epiphysis remains intact. The combination of early adequate incision, adequate antibiotic therapy, and removal of the seques-

205

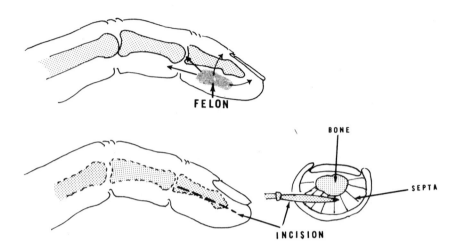

FIGURE 155. Felon, pulp abscess. A pulp infection may spread in the direction shown by the arrows—to the tip, to the dorsum, or retrograde into the distal joint or the flexor tendon sheath. The pulp is divided into compartments by vertical septa. Incision for a felon must cut across these septa and be near the nail to avoid later scarring of the sensitive tactile surface.

trum will give good results. Whenever possible, early referral to a hand surgeon should be made for definitive care.

Paronychia

Paronychia is an infection that occurs on the dorsum of the distal digit at the base of the nail (Fig. 156). Initially, there is redness, pain, and swelling. It is usually sufficient to elevate the skin fold over the base of the nail and incise into the sulcus along the side of the nail. If the infection has spread under the nail, it may be necessary to remove the base of the nail and pack under the remaining skin flap.

Fascia and Tendon Sheaths

Figure 157 shows the direction and site of incision for draining infections in the fascial spaces. Most infections are palmar, but they spread and swell on the dorsum of the hand since the dorsal tissues are looser. Most incisions for drainage, therefore, are made on the palmar surface. The site of the infection is located at the area of maximum tenderness, local heat, and swelling. Usually, infections are contained in the midpalmar space, the ulnar or radial bursal areas, or the thenar space. The various areas of localized infection are beyond the scope of this presentation, but several cardinal principles must be observed.

206

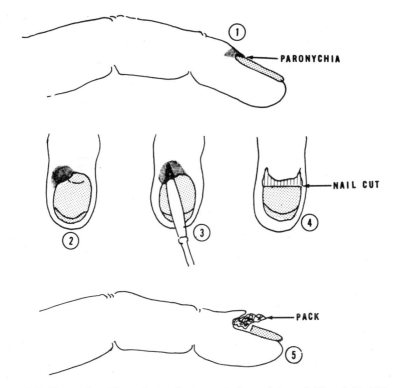

FIGURE 156. Paronychia. This infection begins at the base of the nail (1) and (2). If found early, it may be treated by elevating the overhanging skin by a sharp probe (3) and releasing the pus. If infection is too severe, the nail may be cut (4); the proximal nail is removed exposing the bed, and elevating and packing under the overhanging skin (5) are done.

When an infection spreads into the tendon sheaths of the second, third, or fourth fingers, drainage is accomplished by incising along the lateral aspect of the fingers. The incision must be made dorsal to the finger creases (see Fig. 157) to avoid cutting the digital nerves and arteries. Incision of the fifth finger is made on its radial side because less friction and trauma occur on that side. For the same reason, incision is made on the ulnar side of the second (index) finger.

A midpalmar incision (see Fig. 157) is made along or slightly proximal to the distal palmar crease. Once the palmar aponeurosis is penetrated, unusual care must be exercised to visualize and avoid injuring the digital branches of the median and ulnar nerves deep in the palm.

Drainage of a thenar abscess is done by incision on the *dorsum* of the web space between the thumb and index finger parallel to the margin of the web. If an incision is made on the palmar aspect of the thumb and thenar space, the proximal extent of the incision must be curtailed to

207

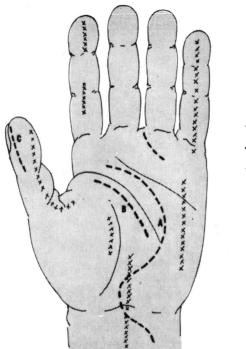

FIGURE 157. Site of incision for hand infections. (A) Incision for drainage of the palmar space between the median and ulnar nerves. The incision curves across the wrist crease to avoid contracture. (B) The incision for draining the thenar space parallels the thenar crease. (C) The incision for drainage of felon transects fascial planes and avoids tactile surfaces. Cutting should be avoided *across* creases, over nerves and blood vessels, and through tactile surfaces.

avoid cutting the motor branch of the median nerve to the thenar muscles.

Infection that spreads into flexor tendon sheaths displays Kanavel's[1] four cardinal signs: (1) finger held in slight flexion, (2) uniform swelling along the tendon sheath (as compared with localized swelling in the typical carbuncle), (3) intense pain on attempting to extend the finger, and (4) tenderness along the *entire* course of the tendon.

Principles of Treatment

It is apparent that proper care of hand infections requires combined use of local heat applications, elevation of the hand, proper use of specific antibiotics, resting the part in the physiologic position of function, and incising for drainage. The latter requires extensive knowledge of anatomic structures.

Any surgery done on the hand must be undertaken under strict sterile conditions, preferably in an operating room and under ideal anesthesia. A bloodless field gives excellent exposure and is ensured by wrapping the entire extremity with an elastic dressing, then using a blood pressure cuff inflated to 250 mm of mercury as a preferred tourniquet.

Unusual infections such as anthrax, gonorrhea, syphilis, tuberculosis, and various mycoses are suspected by their clinical appearance and must be verified by appropriate laboratory procedures. They respond to the fundamental care of all infections supplemented by specific antibiotic or chemotherapeutic drugs.

VASCULAR IMPAIRMENT

Vascular impairment of the upper extremity can result from trauma, infection, or occlusive disease. The latter may variably evolve from embolic, thrombotic, neural, thermal, or mechanical pressure factors. The end result of vascular impairment is tissue necrosis with scarring, loss of muscle and tendon functions, nerve impairment, and joint contracture.

Raynaud's Phenomenon

This condition is attributed to arterial spasm usually triggered by cold or emotional stress. It is most prevalent in women, occurs around age 40, and usually is experienced bilaterally. An episode consists of sudden pallor of the fingers, which may progress to complete blanching. The initial vasospastic period is followed by cyanosis, then a reflex vasodilatation in which the hand becomes hyperemic. Gangrene is rare.

Raynaud's phenomenon is a manifestation of vasomotor instability with abnormal sympathetic response to stress. This response may be secondary to numerous problems of the uncommonly recognized *cervical dorsal outlet syndrome* (anterior scalene syndrome, pectoralis minor, or claviculocostal syndromes). Raynaud's phenomenon may be the forerunner of manifest collagen vascular disease such as scleroderma. It may result from repetitive occupational trauma such as operation of a pneumatic drill. Regardless of the cause, nicotine is considered to be an aggravating drug.

Treatment should attack the cause and simultaneously support the susceptible patient with reassurance and prophylactic advice. Regardless of the cause, smoking *must* be discontinued. In inclement weather, warm clothing and gloves must be worn. Handling iced objects must be avoided. Therapeutic drugs for the increase of arterial circulation, such as nicotinic acid or priscoline, are sometimes advocated, but they give only temporary relief. In severe cases, sympathectomy may be necessary.

209

Raynaud's phenomenon may result from mechanical neurovascular compression of the brachial plexus and the subclavian artery. Such compression may result from an anomalous first rib or a large cervical rib with or without contracted scalene musculature. Pressure upon the artery may cause thromboembolic disease with occlusion. Surgical exploration of the subclavian artery is necessary, along with resection of the cervical or anomalous first rib.

The vasospastic disease described by Burger[2] rarely affects the upper extremity.

Disturbances Due to Cold

The impairment resulting from the exposure of the hand to extremes of cold varies with the extent of low temperature, the duration of the exposure, the presence or absence of moisture and air movement, and the premorbid condition of the patient. Injury is more prevalent in a person with vasomotor instability, general debility, the habit of tobacco use, and underlying vascular disease or previous regional trauma.

Chilblains is a mild cutaneous reaction from repeated exposure of dry skin to temperatures ranging from freezing to 60°F (0° to 15.56°C). The skin becomes red, warm, swollen, and itchy, but there is no tissue destruction. Treatment consists of avoidance of exposure with proper clothing. Soothing ointments may be used for subjective comfort.

Frostbite resembles first- and second-degree burns in its depth of tissue involvement. First-degree frostbite causes redness of the skin followed by desquamation. Second-degree frostbite undergoes blistering followed by desquamation. Frostbite usually occurs from a brief exposure to extreme cold—below 20°F (−7°C). The skin suddenly blanches, may tingle, then becomes anesthetic, and is brittle.

Frostbite must be thawed immediately by immersion in a water bath of 104° to 109°F (40° to 42.78°C). A whirlpool, when available, is excellent treatment. When hydrotherapy is not available, the hand or hands can be placed under clothing into the opposite axilla. The frostbitten hand must never be rubbed or covered with snow or slush.

Antibiotics should be started early. The hands are then wrapped in nonadhesive gauze and placed in firm pressure dressings. Active motion of the hand and fingers should be avoided, since the tissues are often brittle; such motions cause the skin to crack. Sympathectomy and anticoagulation therapy have been disappointing.

The depth of tissue injury determines the extent of residual impairment. Blisters usually occur within 24 to 36 hours and the skin blackens within 10 to 14 days. The exact mechanism of tissue destruction is currently unknown. Crystals form within the tissues, but the site and source of these crystals are obscure. As the frozen tissues thaw, lymph flow increases, as does capillary permeability, and edema results. Superficial blebs occur, along with varying degrees of tissue necrosis.

Rapid thawing done *in the field* where the tissues may be refrozen should be avoided. Refreezing of tissues invariably ends in gangrene. Drinking alcohol to increase circulation defeats its purpose by the cooling effect of peripheral dilatation. The *general* body temperature must be elevated.

Occlusive Vascular Diseases

Occlusive vascular diseases may occur from embolic fragments originating from proximal thrombus formation, as in rheumatic heart disease. Vascular anomalies and post-traumatic arteriovenous fistula may impair distal arterial circulation. Arteriography and appropriate surgery must be undertaken. Early referral to a hand surgeon or a vascular surgeon can salvage the impaired hand.

Volkmann's ischemic contracture results from vascular occlusion at the level of the elbow or forearm—most commonly the result of unexpected swelling in a plaster cast or from vascular compromise following a fracture or dislocation of the elbow. Other forms of trauma may cause this condition, such as fractures of the forearm bones, hematomas from penetrating wounds, prolonged application of tourniquets, or even prolonged pressure upon the forearm during an alcoholic stupor.

Pressure most often affects the flexor compartment of the forearm because of its peculiar anatomic structure. The compartment is tightly bound at all its attachments and cannot expand to accommodate increased internal pressure. Pressure within this compartment from edema, venous congestion, or hemorrhage causes ischemic necrosis of the muscle, tendon, and nerve tissue.

The onset may be catastrophically abrupt with sudden painful swelling and discoloration of the forearm and hand. Cyanosis, coldness, and numbness are noted early. If pressure persists, there may be necrosis of the flexors of the wrist and hand. The extensors are usually spared. The median and ulnar nerves are frequently involved, but the radial nerve escapes entrapment.

The resultant deformity from this ischemic contracture is hyperextension of the metacarpophalangeal joints (resulting from unopposed extensors) and flexion contracture of the interphalangeal and wrist joints (owing to the contracted flexor muscles). The forearm is atrophic, and a typical median-ulnar nerve hand results.

The best treatment is prevention. A constrictive cast must be released as soon as it is recognized. Elbow fractures or dislocations, or both, must be promptly and properly reduced. When done expeditiously, these measures usually ensure proper circulation.

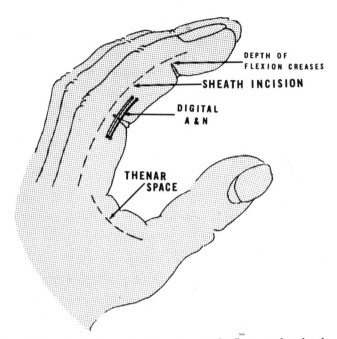

DEPTH OF
FLEXION CREASES

SHEATH INCISION

DIGITAL
A & N

THENAR
SPACE

FIGURE 158. Incisions for sheath infection. Incisions in the flexor tendon sheaths are made on the radial side of the fifth finger and the ulnar side of the second finger. The incision must be dorsal to the depth of the flexion crease to avoid the digital nerve and blood vessels. Infection of the thenar space is drained by a dorsal incision parallel to the margin of the web between the thumb and index finger.

When circulation appears compromised from significant swelling of the forearm, pressure should be relieved by splitting the muscle fascia along the full length of the muscle bellies. The incision should be allowed to gape. The incision should angle at the bend of the elbow and all the major blood vessels should be viewed and freed from any obstruction. A skin graft should then cover the incision to avoid direct, open exposure of the underlying muscles. The arm and hand should be elevated and the fingers and wrist splinted in a physiologic position. Early sympathectomy improves the circulation.

Any hand impairment resulting from ischemic contracture should be treated extensively by conservative measures before constructive surgery is contemplated. Serial stretch splints to extend the deforming contractures should be applied and changed frequently as increased range of motion is gained. These should be used for several months, exercising care to protect the skin from unrelieved pressure. Physical therapy consisting of active and passive exercises supplemented by occupational therapy must be continued throughout the period of splinting and after the splinting has achieved its ultimate gains. This type of therapy should be employed

212

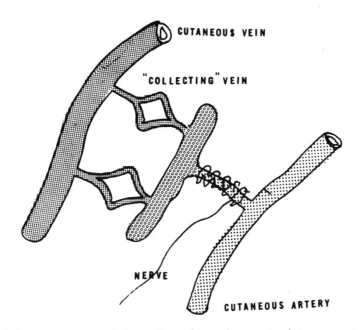

CUTANEOUS VEIN

"COLLECTING" VEIN

NERVE

CUTANEOUS ARTERY

FIGURE 159. Glomus tumor. The tumor is an abnormal connection between a cutaneous artery and vein in which there is swelling and thus irritation of the sensory unmyelinated nerve of the collecting arterioles.

preoperatively and postoperatively, once reconstructive surgery is contemplated.

Vascular impairment of the hand also includes Sudeck's atrophy, reflex sympathetic dystrophy, shoulder-hand syndrome, minor and major causalgias, and so forth. These topics have been covered in previous chapters.

GLOMUS TUMORS

A glomus tumor is a tiny, subungual, painful tumor. The normal glomus is essentially an arteriovenous anastomosis without an intermediary capillary bed. The tumor is a "caricature" of the normal neuromyoarterial glomus with hypertrophy of the normal glomus elements. Myelinated and unmyelinated nerve fibers terminate within the glomus (Fig. 159). Grossly, the tumor is soft, and pink or purple, its defined elongated mass the size of a grain of rice.

The symptoms of a glomus tumor are pain, tenderness, and external sensitivity to temperature (cold more than heat). The mass (glomus) becomes visible or palpable after a considerable period of time, so symptoms can be present long before it is evident. When the tumor becomes visible, it may appear as a blue spot in the subungual region, and there may be

213

deforming ridges in the nail with the lesion being exquisitely tender. Subjectively, the pain is termed sharp and cutting (lancinating).

Treatment consists of complete surgical removal. It may be necessary to remove the nail completely, shell out the lesion meticulously, and currette down to bleeding bone.

ENVENOMATION (SNAKEBITES)

Snakebites frequently affect the hand. There are four families of snakes that inject venom that may be neurotonic or hematonic. The elapid snakes (corals, cobras, mambas) emit primarily neurotonic venom; vipers (rattlesnakes, water moccasins, copperheads) inject chiefly hematonic venom. Snakebites from all these varieties produce cardiac, respiratory, and hematologic changes with some degree of central nervous affliction. The severity of damage done by envenomation depends on the age and size of the patient, depth of the bite, amount of venom injected, size and species of snake, and, most importantly, the quality of first aid and medical care administered.

Signs and Symptoms

The local effects of a venom bite are swelling and pain within 30 minutes. Within several hours, ecchymosis with discoloration appears. Bullae may form at the site within 24 hours. Systemic effects are tingling of lips, tongue, fingers, and toes. Weakness, a faint feeling, and nausea may occur.

Treatment

Within 30 minutes, a tourniquet must be applied 2 to 4 inches proximal to the bite or proximal to the advancing edema. The tourniquet must be tight enough only to occlude the superficial venom circulation. Incision and suction are helpful, but must be performed within minutes of the envenomation and it must be to the depth of the snakebite (fang depth).

The victim must remain physically inactive and receive no alcohol or stimulants. The injured extremity (hand and arm) should be immobilized in a physiologic position and elevated above the heart level. When available, polyvalent antivenom serum should be given, but only in a medical facility in the case of a severe allergic reaction.

When hemorrhagic bullae appear in the hand, they are usually debrided four to six days after the bite has occurred.

Approximately four to seven days after occurrence of a bite, if the general condition of the patient allows it, gentle active and passive range-of-motion exercises of all joints are begun. Because edema may limit the range at this point, elevation and passive movement, as well as gentle massage (to tolerance), are begun. Upon completion of what can be considered the subacute phase—seven days or more—active rehabilitation is begun.

REFERENCES

1. Kanavel, A. B.: Infections of the Hand, ed. 7. Lea, Philadelphia, 1939.
2. Burger, L.: The Circulatory Disturbances of the Extremities. W. B. Saunders, Philadelphia, 1924.

BIBLIOGRAPHY

Allen, E. V. and Brown, G. E.: Raynaud's disease: A clinical study of 147 cases. J.A.M.A. 99:1472, 1932.

Boyes, J. H.: Bunnel's Surgery of the Hand, ed. 4. J. B. Lippincott, Philadelphia, 1964.

Carroll, R. E. and Berman, A. T.: Glomus tumors of the hand. J. Bone Joint Surg. 54-A:697, 1972.

Lampe, E. W.: Surgical anatomy of the hand. Clin. Symp. vol. 9, 1957.

Murray, A. R.: The management of the infected hand: Based on clinical investigation of 513 cases. Med. J. Aust. 1:619, 1951.

Swinton, N. W., et al.: Unilateral Raynaud's phenomenon caused by cervical-first rib anomalies. Am. J. Med. 48:404, 1970.

Wilkinson, J. L.: The anatomy of an oblique proximal septum of the pulp space. Br. J. Surg. 38:454, 1950-51.

215

CHAPTER 10

Splinting the Hand

Proper splinting requires evaluation of impaired hand function, then determination of the exact part to be splinted and the specific objective to be accomplished. The objective sought by splinting determines the type of splint to be used and specifies the duration and frequency of its application.

TYPES OF SPLINTS

A splint can be classified as static, semidynamic, or dynamic. Other terms may be used and other classifications have also been enumerated. These three basic splints fulfill the following functions:

1. Stabilize (immobilize) joints in a desired position to *rest* the joint, tendons, ligaments, and muscles, or maintain a certain bone alignment.
2. Prevent contracture or deformity.
3. Prevent unwanted motion.
4. Gradually stretch contracture to increase range of joint motion.
5. Substitute lost muscle function.
6. Maintain gains achieved by manipulation, corrective surgery, or reconstructive procedures.
7. Relieve pain.

Static

A static splint prevents motion and thus rests the parts indicated. Unfortunately, in accomplishing this purpose this type of splint can also cause disuse atrophy, weakness, stiffness, and dependency. It should never be used longer than is physiologically indicated, and should never be used if a dynamic or semidynamic splint is equally effective. The splint should immobilize *only* the intended joints, leaving all adjacent joints free to move. A resting splint should have smooth surfaces and should be molded accurately to fit properly and to avoid unwanted pressures on bony prominences or nerve areas.

Plaster casts should not be applied circularly, but should be laid on in flat slabs, preferably leaving half of the hand uncovered by plaster. When complete enclosure is necessary, the cast should be bivalved as soon as possible.

Semidynamic

This splint permits no movement, but functions by positioning the parts to perform at their optimum. For example, the thumb carpometacarpal joint can be splinted in abduction-opposition to facilitate pinch grip with the index finger. A semidynamic splint does not use extrinsic power sources such as rubber bands, springs, and so forth.

Dynamic

A dynamic (functional or kinetic) splint can permit, guide, prevent, and actively create or resist certain movements. By necessity there is some degree of hinging and some source of power. Intrinsic power utilizes the patient's own muscles, whereas extrinsic power uses rubber bands, tension wires, springs, or even electronic or pneumatic units. Dynamic splints are used to overcome gravity, correct muscle imbalance, and prevent and correct contracture, thus improving range of motion. These splints may offer resistance for active exercise.

Restoration of function by mechanical extrinsically-powered units is still in an experimental stage. Elaborate power units are being developed constantly and engineering technologic skills are joining with medical research in this endeavor. These advances are beyond the scope of this text but are well documented by Licht[1] and by Anderson.[2]

CONSTRUCTION OF THE SPLINT

Many materials are available for splinting and bracing, each with specific advocates and each with individual advantages. Currently available are varieties of plaster, plastics, nylon fabrics, and metals for splint construction with instructions from the manufacturers.

Construction of the splint requires imagination on the part of the prescriber or the orthotist. Patterns and molds are guidelines and should be modified to meet the special problem. Materials available are numerous and constantly changing. It behooves a frequent user of splinting materials and techniques to become familiar and adept with a special material and then improve a technique while employing new materials as they become available.

Splints should be simple to apply and to use. They should be lightweight, durable, comfortable, easy to keep clean, and cosmetically acceptable to the patient. Specific instructions should be given the wearer concerning the duration and frequency of its use. Activities involving precise movements should be performed while wearing the splint and during the withdrawal of the splint.

Attachment of splints to the hand usually requires straps. These straps should never cross a joint or press against a bony prominence. Areas where nerve pressure is possible should be avoided and a splint should never be so tight or constrictive as to cause edema. Many materials for making straps are also available.

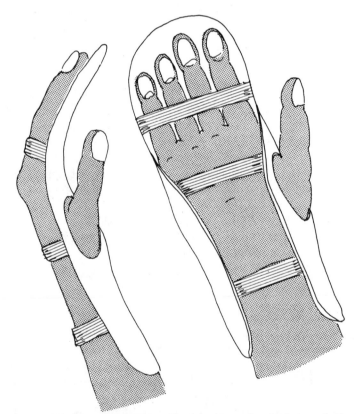

FIGURE 160. Static (rest) splint. This splint can be made of plaster, plastic, Polysar, orthoplast, or other materials and strapped with leather, Velcro, or webbing. It maintains the wrist and fingers in a physiologic position. Among its uses, it is valuable in managing wrist drop from peripheral neuropathies and early flaccid stage of stroke. It prevents deformity, relieves pain, and avoids overstretching of flail musculature.

EXAMPLES OF SPLINTS

Many of the splints mentioned and illustrated in the preceding chapters for specific conditions are not repeated here. The splints depicted in this chapter (Figs. 160-167) are examples of those accepted in current use. In summary, a splint must be created to fulfill specific indications after functional evaluation of the hand and determination of the objective to be accomplished by splinting.

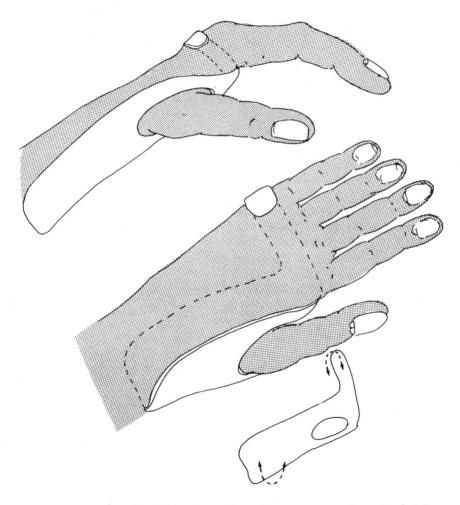

FIGURE 161. Wrist rest splint. This splint can be used as a rest or a semidynamic splint. Its purpose is to maintain the wrist in slight extension, yet permit and assist finger and thumb movement. It can be made of any material. It has definite value in treating median nerve compression (carpal tunnel syndrome).

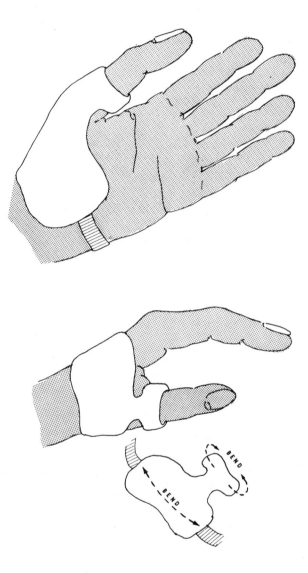

FIGURE 162. Semidynamic thumb splint. This splint is valuable in a flail thumb or in degenerative painful arthritis of the carpometacarpal joint. It immobilizes the thumb in abduction and opposition, permitting tip-to-tip pinch. It has value in spasticity (cerebral palsy), in treating thumb-in-palm, or adducted thumb position.

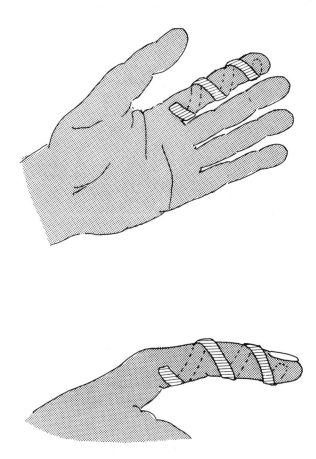

FIGURE 163. Finger rest splint. This simple wrap-around splint uses flexible or plastic material to rest a finger or to maintain gained range of motion in contracture. It provides rest in post-traumatic or degenerative joint changes.

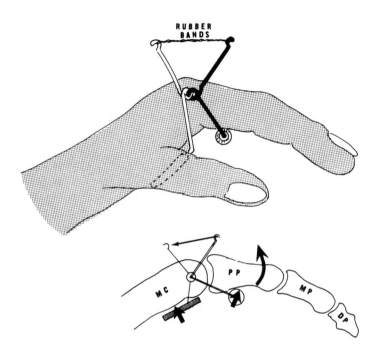

FIGURE 164. Dynamic splint. This type of dynamic splint extends the metacarpophalangeal joint(s). By the power pull of the rubber bands, the proximal phalanx is extended on the metacarpal. There is constant pull while it is being worn. This splint can be used to exercise and strengthen the proximal flexors.

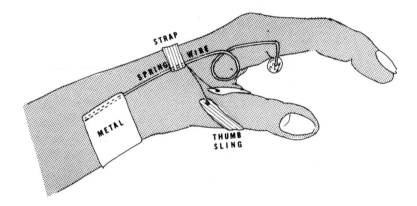

FIGURE 165. Dynamic splint for wrist drop, radial nerve palsy. Using spring wire as a power source, this simple splint extends the wrist and simultaneously abducts the thumb. It is used in radial nerve or nerve root palsies.

222

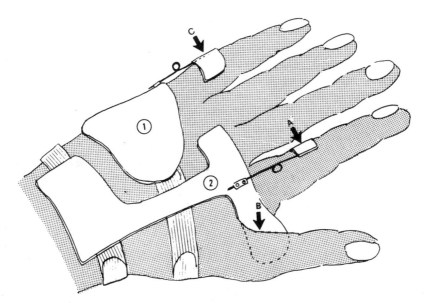

FIGURE 166. Composite dynamic splint, first dorsal interosseous *(A)*, fifth adduction *(C)*. Two spring-wire splints are shown. One *(1)* adducts the fifth finger and another *(2)* assists the first dorsal interosseous-index abduction. *(B)* A flange abducts the thumb. Usually, only one of these splints is worn, or both can be incorporated into one wristband.

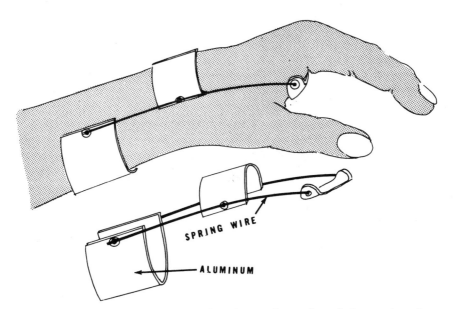

FIGURE 167. Dynamic wrist-drop splint. This splint can be simply made from spring wire and molded aluminum and is an example of the numerous materials that can be employed in making splints.

223

REFERENCES

1. Licht, S. (ed.): Othotics Etcetera (Physical Medicine Library, Vol. 9). Elizabeth Licht Publisher, New Haven, 1966.
2. Anderson, M.: Functional Bracing of the Upper Extremities. Charles C Thomas, Springfield, Ill., 1958.

BIBLIOGRAPHY

Boyes, J. H.: Bunnell's Surgery of the Hand, ed. 4. J. B. Lippincott, Philadelphia, 1964.

Bunnell, S.: The knuckle bender splint. U. S. Army Med. Bull., Feb., 1946.

Bunnell, S.: Splinting the Hand. American Academy of Orthopedic Surgery Instructional Course Lecture, 9:233, 1952.

Redford, J. B., Gilewich, G., and Jiminez, J.: Simple Splints, Principles and Techniques. University of Alberta Hospital, Canada, 1969.

Wynn Parry, C. B.: Rehabilitation of the Hand. Butterworths, London, 1966.

Index

A *t* indicates a table.
An italic page number indicates a figure.

225

Dystrophy, reflex sympathetic, 102–109

ELBOW, muscles about, *21*
Envenomation, 214–215
Evaluation of functional impairment of hand, 168–172
Extension, loss of, 171–172
Extensor apparatus of finger, 39, *38*
Extensor assistant supinator nerve, 25
Extensor carpi ulnaris, ulnar subluxation of, *154*
Extensor digital mechanism, 39–42
Extensor digiti quinti proprius, *80*
Extensor digitorum communis, *80*
Extensor forearm muscles, 21–22, *20*
Extensor indicis proprius, *83*
Extensor lateral bands, *41*
Extensor of metacarpophalangeal joint, *43*
Extensor pollicis brevis, *83*
Extensor pollicis longus
    rupture of, 118, *118*
Extensor tendon, *44*
    pull, *40*
    rupture at middle phalanx, 115–118
    severance of, 111–112
Extrinsic muscles, 19–32

FELON infection, 205–206, *206*
Fiberglas splint, burns and, 199, *200*
Finger(s). *See also* Hand.
    burns of, 197–204
    changes in shoulder-hand-finger syndrome, *107*
    edema of,
        dorsal, 107–108
            treatment of, 108–109
            removal of, 108, 109, *109*
    extensor apparatus of, 39, *38*
    fractures and dislocations of, 128–143
    infections of, 205–215
    joints, injuries to and diseases of, 144–178
    movement of
        controlling factor in, 27
        functional, 35, *36*
    nerve control of, 50–100
    positioning during hemiplegia, *183*
    reflex sympathetic dystrophy of, 102–109
    rest splint, *221*
    shoulder-hand-finger syndrome, 106–109
    spasticity, 180–196
    splints, 216–223

tendinous insertion into, 25–32
tendons, injuries to and diseases of, 111–126
Finger spreader approximator nerve, 25
Flexion, loss of, 171–172
Flexor carpi radialis, *13, 25, 59*
Flexor carpi ulnaris, 72, *72*
Flexor digiti minimi muscle, 48
Flexor digitorum profundus, 72, *63, 73*
Flexor digitorum sublimis, *61*
Flexor forearm muscles, 22–25
Flexor pollicis brevis muscle, 46, *67*
Flexor pollicis longus, *13, 25, 62*
Flexor pronator thumb-finger approximator nerve, 25
Flexor tendinous insertion into digits, 25–32, *26*
Flexor tendon
    rupture of, 119
    severance of, 112–113
Fracture(s)
    Bennett, 136–137, *137*
    carpal scaphoid bone, 142, *141*
    Colles', 140–143, *138, 139, 140*
    healing time, *131*
    hematoma in, *131*
    metacarpal, 136
        base of fifth, 137–138
        neck, *134*
    middle phalanx, 134–135
    phalangeal, mechanism of deformation, *130*
    principles of treatment of, 128–132
        immobilization of finger joints in, *129*
        plaster traction in, *132*
    scaphoid bone, 142, *141*
    terminal phalanx, 133
    thumb, 136–137, *135, 137*
    wrist, 140–143
Friction
    flexor tendons and, 26
Froment's sign, positive in ulnar nerve paralysis, 75
Frostbite, 210–211
Functional impairment
    evaluation of, 168–172
Functional position of hand, 87

GLOMUS tumors, 213–214, *213*
Grip(s)
    hook, *35*
    key, 170, *169*

227

228

sprains of, 144–146
"stiffness of," 19

KEY grip, 170, *169*

LESIONS
median nerve, 64–70
radial nerve, 77–80
ulnar nerve, 76–77
Ligament(s). *See also* Articulation(s);
  Joint(s).
  collateral, 5
  of Henle, 6
  intercarpal, 8, *7*
  intermetacarpal, 19
  metacarpophalangeal, *158*
  oblique, 5, 6
  oblique retinacular, contracture of, 126,
    125
  transverse, 5, 6
  'transverse carpal, 10–11, *11*
  transverse metacarpal, *18*
  wrist, 5–8, *6*
Lumbrical muscles, 35–39
  nerve compression and, 87
Lunate, 7
Lunate carpal bone dislocation, *147*

MALLET finger, 165, *164*
  causes of, 114, *114*
  treatment for, 114–115
    plaster cast, *115*
    rationale for, *115*
Median nerve, *13, 25, 51, 57, 65*
  anatomy of, 58–63
  cervical root component, *70*
  compression in, 86–92, *91*
    treatment of, 90, 92
  control of hand, 25, 58–63
  damage to, 56
  pronator teres syndrome in, 91–92
    treatment of, 92
  root lesion of, 65–70
  severance of, 64–65, 82–83
    testing for, 80
    treatment of, 85–86
Metacarpal, injury to, 136–138
Metacarpal bones
  alignment of, *155*
  anatomy of, 14–15
Metacarpal joint, *48, 157*
Metacarpophalangeal articulations, 15–19
Metacarpophalangeal joints,

extensor of, *43*
normal flexion-extension of, *108*
subluxation of, *145*
volar subluxation of, 160, *161*
Metacarpophalangeal ligaments, *158*
Motor neuron disease, upper, 180–196
Muscle(s). *See also* specific muscles.
  changes in
    nerve lesions and, 56
    nerve severance and, 56
  dorsal group, 25
  extensor assistant supinator group, 25
  extensor forearm, 21–22
  extrinsic, anatomy of, 19–32
  extrinsic finger, 27–32
  flexor carpi radialis, 11
  flexor carpi ulnaris, 5, 11
  flexor forearm, 22–25
  flexor pronator group, 25
  hand, 5
  hypothenar group, 48–49, *46, 47*
  interossei, 34–35, 36–37, 39, *32, 33*
  intrinsic, *34*
    anatomy of, 33–49
    of the thenar and hypothenar groups,
      42–49
  lumbrical, 35–36, 37–39
    nerve compression and, 87
  palmar group, 25
  spasm, ulnar drift and, *159*
  terminology for, 25
  thenar group, 42–46, *46, 47*
  voluntary, testing of, 55
Musculature of thenar eminence, *69*

NERVE(s). *See also* specific nerves.
  compression, 86–98
  control of hand, 50–100
  damage
    degrees of, 55–56
    muscle changes following, 56
  injury, degrees of, *54*
  median. *See* Median nerve.
  peripheral. *See* Peripheral nerve.
  radial. *See* radial nerve.
  root, 52
  severance, 50–86
    sensory tests and, 50–55
    Weber test and, 51–52
  terminology for, 25
  ulnar. *See* Ulnar nerve.
Neurotmesis, 56
"No man's land," 112–113, *113*

229